Sensation: Intelligibility in Sensibility

Contemporary Studies in Philosophy and the Human Sciences

Series Editors:
Hugh J. Silverman and Graeme Nicholson

Published

Forthcoming

* **Available in paperback**

Sensation:
Intelligibility in
Sensibility

———◆———

Alphonso Lingis

HUMANITIES PRESS
NEW JERSEY

First published in 1996 by Humanities Press International Inc.,
165 First Avenue, Atlantic Highlands, New Jersey 07716

©1996 by Alphonso Lingis

Library of Congress Cataloging-in-Publication Data
Lingis, Alphonso
 Sensation : intelligibility in sensibility / Alphonso Lingis.
  p. cm.—(Contemporary studies in philosophy and the human
 scienses)
 Includes index.
 ISBN 0–391–03899–0
 1. Sense (Philosophy) 2. Senses and sensation. 3. Perception (Philosophy)
 4. Phenomenology—Controversial literature. 5. Existentialism—Controversial
 literature. I. Title.
 II. Series.
 B105.S45L56 1996   95–21456
 121'.3—dc20   CIP

Printed in the United States of America

Contents

◆

The condition of pleasure called intoxication is precisely an exalted feeling of *power*—The sensations of space and time are altered: tremendous distances are surveyed and, as it were, for the first time apprehended; the extension of vision over greater masses and expanses; the refinement of the organs for the apprehension of much that is extremely small and fleeting: *divination*, the power of understanding with only the least assistance, at the slightest suggestion: "intelligent" *sensuality*—; strength as a feeling of dominion in the muscles, as suppleness and pleasure in movement, as dance, as levity and *presto*; strength as pleasure in the proof of strength, as bravado, adventure, fearlessness, indifference to life or death—All these climactic moments of life mutually stimulate one another; the world of images and ideas of the one suffices as a suggestion for the others—in this way, states finally merge into one another though they might have good reason to remain apart.

—Friedrich Nietzsche, *The Will to Power*, ¶800

List of Illustrations

———◆———

Photographs are by the author.

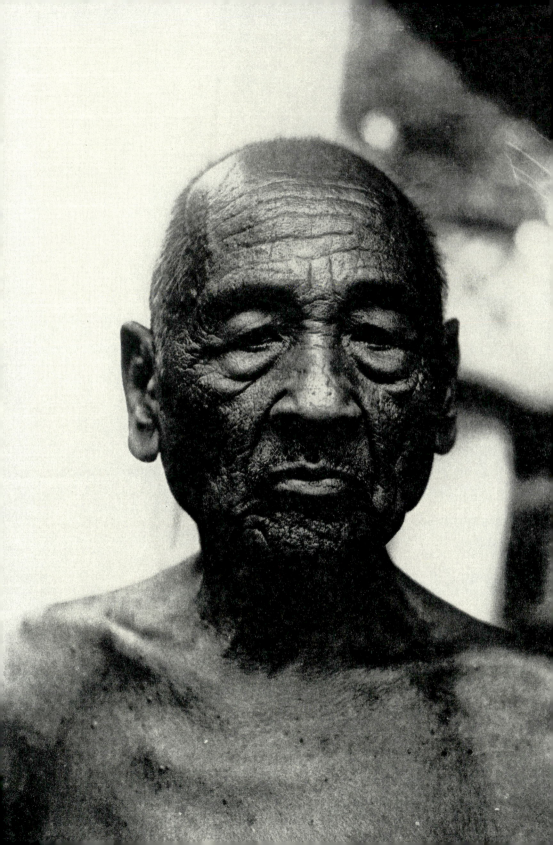

Foreword

◆

The studies in this book question theses which existential philosophy has derived out of its phenomenological investigations. Phenomenology is a descriptive elaboration of the field of consciousness. It takes the phenomenal field of which we are conscious in the perceptual, affective, and practical activities of life to be the primary layout of reality. The field of which we are conscious is not an inner psychic representation whose index of reality corresponds to the reality of our sensations. Phenomenology argues that our sensations themselves are intentional; they are givens of sense, or give sense—orientation and meaning. In the course of questioning the theses phenomenology has given rise to, we find ourselves advancing toward a new notion of what sensation, sensibility, sensuality, and susceptibility are, and a new notion of the intelligence in them.

We find problems in the way negativity has entered phenomenological descriptions. Existential philosophy admitted an experience of nothingness, involved in our sense of being mortal. The most negative experience, experience of nothingness itself, was then shown to convert into the most positive experience, positing my existence as my own and positing the world in its totality. This dialectical strain in existential thinking seems unreliable to us.

Can dying be identified as the passage from being to nothingness? Can death be identified as nothingness? Is it the fear in the sense of one's own mortality that makes one not equivalent to and interchangeable with others? Does the anxiety that senses one's own death singling one out singularize one? Does the existence that anticipates its own end makes possible the unilateral determination of means to determinate ends in the field before one? Is having-to-die the imperative that makes imperative all the imperatives that thought and action recognize?

Every human experience is not only in the world, existential philosophy declared, but is an experience of the world. Unlike animals who exist in their environments, we exist in the world. The notion that our apprehension of things presupposes a comprehensive grasp of the context—and that this context is the world—this holistic strain in phenomenology seems to us to be open to question.

Does the comprehensive grasp of the whole practicable field precede and make possible the determination of an implement? Is the world the context in which practical action takes form? Are instrumental connections the underlying order of the real world that link up the practicable fields of our discontinuous and limited initiatives? Does an emotion, turned to an object or situation, arise on the ground of a mood, which senses how one is subjected to the world? How are both the instrumental layout envisioned in practical action and the weight of the landscape sensed in mood identified as the world? Do moods obturate our view, absorb us in the immediacy of things? Does the sense of mortality, which singularizes an agent, disconnect him or her from the myopic absorption in everyday situations, and open him or her upon the world? Does the sense of the nothingness of death give us a sense of the world, suspended contingently in the abyss?

Existential philosophy also promoted a holistic conception to overcome the conflict between perception, feeling, and action. In fact our sentient bodies do withdraw from the integrated praktognostic orientation to things and sink into monocular images, pre-things, phantasms, twilight and fog. The phenomenology of perception claimed to find in perceptual life a teleological orientation to the perception of integrated intersensorial things, to praktognostic competence, and an imperative orientation to a coherent and consistent world. We find also other imperatives, imperative incompetence and imperative letting go of the world. The phenomenology of perception promoted an intentional and structural conception of the sensory-motor body. We set out to recover a substantive conception of our bodies given to excitement and lust.

Is every consciousness consciousness of something? Is a figure against a background the structure of all perception? What is the imperative in things, and the imperative that we have to perceive things? Is the constancy of the normal, right, or true properties of the things we perceive explainable by the coherence and consistency of the world? Does our access to the world explain our tendency to entrench ourselves in phantasms? Is then the world not given in perception, but imperative?

Is the theoretical objective, to represent the things we observe as objects and the field opened by our perception as an objective universe, itself motivated by the structure of things which command our perception? Are the concepts and forms of organization science admits into its objective representation of the universe derived from perception? Is the perceived world the real in which all regions objectively represented by scientific disciplines have to be situated?

Is perception a praktognosis; is it directed upon objectives? Is perceptual competence practical competence? Does incompetence signify disconnection from the real?

Phenomenology took experience to be from the first consciousness of a figure against a background; it showed that the figure is a meaningful intersensorial pattern, a lure or repellant, and a reachable and manipulatable objective, and that the background is structured with significant instrumental connections and affectively charged. What perceives is the whole sensory-motor body, and the postural schema that integrates its movements integrates its receptor surfaces. We have found this primacy of praktognostic perception idealist and this contextualist conception of sensation doubtful.

What is the relationship between sensation as apprehension of the sense— the orientation and meaning—of things and sensation as sensual contact with them? Is sensuality intentional? If posture is the *sensus communis* that integrates our receptor surfaces and gives us a perception of an intersensorial thing, what happens when sensual excitement arises in the compulsion to break up the stable organization of skills and competencies? Does the body image that taking up a posture produces give us a sense of our bodies not as diagrams of force but as substances? How explain that the body's knowing that converges its sensitive surfaces upon things and contracts their postures turns to pursuit, penetration, detachment, dismemberment, and dissection of them? What is the relationship between pleasure in equilibrium and in competence and excitement? Is sensual excitement masochist? Or does the excitement in shattering established structures that made resistance, defense, and domination possible anticipate more advanced, more integrated structures of competence?

Existential philosophy replaced substance ontology with a relational conception of intramundane things and an intentional conception of the ex-istence of sentient bodies. We think that the phenomenology that emphasized the intentional form of the body in action has to be supplemented with a phenomonology of its substance. Psychoanalysis, which sees in voluptuous pleasure a discharge of excess energies and a return to the quiescence of the inanimate, and phenomenology, which sees in sexual craving a behavior and a specific kind of intentional initiative, both lose sight of the transubstantiation the body undergoes in pleasure.

What is the relationship between the innate reproductive organs and processes and drive that we call sex, and the swarming of nonteleological impulses seeking the pleasure unpleasure of excitement which Freud called libido? What is the relationship between the theater of appearances, adornment, masquerade, simulation, and intrigue by which individuals make themselves attractive to one another, captivate and enslave one another that Baudrillard has identified as seduction, and the corporeal transformation itself—the shattering of the form that frees the substance, and the voluptuous pleasure of this transubstantiation, which we call lust?

Existential philosophy argued not only for the primacy of the world over every private and immanent field of experience, but for the primacy of the common world. The sentient subject is from the first an intersubjectivity. But in this intersubjectivity the other could only be conceived as a variant of oneself, marked by differences. We found this holism contestable. We set out to distinguish between the other as "another one," as "different," and as "other." We then set out to differentiate the common world from the space distended by others in their otherness.

What produces the difference between dealing with another as equivalent and interchangeable with oneself—another one—and dealing with the other as different, situated in another layout of possibilities, in a time nonsimultaneous with one's own? In what does the otherness of the other consist? What is recognizing the other? How does discourse with others have not only indicative and informative form, but vocative and imperative force? How does the I become a seat of responsibility? Do the intentions and foresight of an I measure the extent of his or her responsibility?

Taking every determination to be a negation, existential philosophy, took the apprehension of beings to contain an apprehensiveness about nothingness. The discernment with which I come to see myself as different from others would come from a sense of the singularity of the death coming for me and the nonsimultaneity of my deathbound trajectory of life with those of others. We have not found intelligible this ontology that takes not difference, distance, gradation, and otherness, but being and nothingness to be primitive notions.

Is sensation really a sensitivity for the possible? Does it involve a sense of the impossible? Does it contain a premonition of nothingness? Is the sense of nothingness that which gives us a sense of what is and how far it extends? Does the concern for things contain an apprehensiveness about nothingness—about death? Is there then an exposure to nothingness in the sensitivity with which we are open to the outside environment? What is the relationship between the sensitivity for things and the sensitivity for the sensitivity and sensuality of other sentient beings? Does, as Kant thought, the respect for others mortify our own sensuality? What is the relationship between the space in which we encounter sensible things and the space in which we encounter other sentient beings? What is the relationship between the space in which things are objective or intersubjective, and the field of a perception and action which are my own? Can one affirm that the world is common from the start?

Existential philosophy did not so much show how truth is constituted in discourse as show how speech empties out in communication. The maxim "Back to the things themselves!" called for a reactivation of insight in the first person singular to recover the truth of what got lost sight of in communication. What is said has to be reactivated as what I see and say and answer for. Knowledge requires self-consciousness as an active responsibility. But we think that existential philosophy has not defined or practiced a communication in which the speaker knows how to be authentically responsible.

How is it that I can use an expression in general terms to recall a singular event of my experience, but whenever I communicate with others, the general terms all designate instead recurrent patterns of events? Does not all communication produce loss of insight into the particular, that is, the real? How does communication communicate the difference between interlocutors? Is this difference anything but different intersections of classes and series? What is the nature of the assurance communication brings—is it really an assurance about reality? Or is it an assurance against unreality? In actively and responsibly entering into communication, does not self-consciousness itself empty out? How is self-consciousness a need? Is self-consciousness a means of mastery or of servility? Are one's needs communicable, but one's own powers ineffable? Are words not only forms, that inform, but also forces, that intensify? Can there be a communication that would intensify and consecrate the sensitivity and sensuality of interlocutors?

For existential philosophy, truth is still what is at stake in discourse; discourse was envisioned as the process that articulates and maintains constant the lineaments of the intersubjective world. We have found the philosophy that takes truth to be the supreme value to be questionable.

How can appeals and demands communicated to me have imperative force? Are they not representations whose meaning is reconstituted by me? If I recognize them to have imperative force, are they not laws I legislate for myself? An imperative presents what is not there and what is not me—does its force subsist in a metaphysical realm? Is it something encountered in the phenomenal world? Is the other anything but an exemplar of a law I recognize weighing immediately on my own understanding—or an illustration of it? Does the force of the appeals and demands another addresses to me lie in his or her existence as an ideal, norm, or standard into which I have insight? Why would the figure of another sentient being be the sole locus of an imperative addressed to me? Are there no imperatives that lie in things? Is not all recognition of appeals and demands addressed to me by others a form of pity, which makes me dependent and takes on their wants and needs? What would it mean to communicate with another sovereign one, without needs or wants?

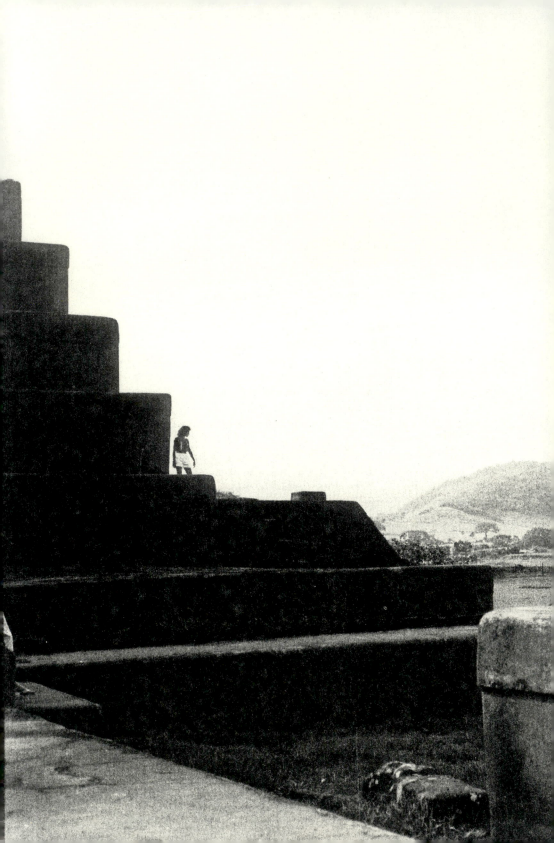

1

♦

We Mortals

One is born with forces that one did not contrive. One lives by giving form to those forces. The forms one gets from the others. One takes one's place in a place another has vacated. One sits in chairs, opens doors, rides a tricycle, one's body catching on how from the others. Chairs, doors, tricycles themselves require and indicate certain postures and movements of one's limbs. They are not made for one's body in particular, but for anyone of a certain age and a certain general size. One makes oneself someone, another one, by taking on the posture and movement they require. Taking a seat in the library, working out the theorems of geometry as they have been worked out by generations of students in this library, one makes oneself a student, another student. Buying another car from the assembly line, paying for it with a check, driving to the supermarket and the disco, one makes oneself a modern westerner. Buying jeans and a business suit, walking in a stride, throwing the baseball with the full thrust of one's torso, sprawling when sitting, one makes one's originally polymorphously perverse infantile body male; buying a dress and lipstick, waving one's fingers, sitting without crossing one's legs, throwing the baseball with only one's arm and not the full torso, one makes one's originally polymorphously perverse infantile body female. One gives one's experiences form by identifying things with the names with which everyone calls them, by seeing the paths and the obstacles others see, by envisioning the goals others are turned to. One says, about the weather, about the boring town and the exciting big city, about the communists, about the football game, about the new album, what one says, what others say. To learn to think is to learn what others think, about physics, about astronomy, about molecular biology, about keeping up one's car, and about managing a business. One learns to see things by following the eyes and gestures of others; one learns to feel solid and flexible and liquid and textured things by manipulating and palpating things as others do. One gives the confusion of sensations and drives in one's head form by

1

feeling about the concert as others feel, by feeling about one's wedding and about funerals as one feels about weddings and funerals, by feeling as one feels, as anyone feels, indignation about social slights and boredom with operas and disgust before pigs and snakes.

One makes oneself someone by giving oneself form. One acquires an identity, a gender, a function, a solidity; one overcomes the malaise and feeling of impotence that accompanies the confused stirring of one's forces and impulses. One makes oneself someone, another one of a series. The forms of one's movements and postures, of one's gaits and gestures, of one's conversations and one's thoughts, and of one's feelings and one's perceptions one picks up from others, passes on to others. One feels oneself a wave on a sea of life that comes indefinitely from the past and extends indefinitely into the future. What one is, one's formed identity, subsists, is there intact every morning after the dissolution of sleep, is there intact every day after years on the job. One feels the consolation of feeling that as the days and the months and the years pass, one's identity does not pass. There is a kind of fear of death that is the undercurrent in all this expenditure of energy to acquire form, a seeking of consolation in the recognition that after years on the job one can still do it as well as the twenty-year-old they just hired, that after so many years in the classroom paid for one's trained brain one can answer the questions each generation of students ask.

In these forms one confines the excesses of force and feeling that sometimes well up in one. One arranges one's home and one's situation and one's workday in such a way that those once-in-a-lifetime situations which would require all of one's forces, forces that may prove wanting, do not occur. One retains, behind the forms of one's routine, a reserve of force, for the tasks that will recur the next day. One retains, behind the forms of one's thought and speech, a reserve of unused mental energy; one settles into an occupation that presents only the tasks that one has already contracted the mental skills for. One avoids confronting issues that would require all of one's mental agility, which may prove wanting; one avoids problems at the farthest limits of mathematics or physics or politics for which no solution has ever been formulated by thinkers and for which one's own mind may prove wanting. One retains, behind the coded forms of one's feelings, one's pleasures and one's angers, one's affections and one's annoyances, a reserve of force, so that one will be able to respond emotionally to like events and like situations that recur. One arranges one's zone of activities and one's travels in such a way as to avoid once-in-a-lifetime situations that would require all one's passion, which might prove wanting. One avoids going to places utterly unlike any other, which would leave one wholly overwhelmed with an astonishment that could never recur again. One immediately compares each city and each landscape and each building with cities and landscapes and buildings one has seen before and others one still sees, so that one can frame one's feeling in the forms and confines of feelings that one can repeat indefinitely. One avoids situations and adventures in which one might be swept away with a total and totally new joy, sensing that one could never know such a joy again. One avoids encounters in which one might fall blindingly in love; one seeks out instead people others might also fall in love with and one loves one's partner as others love like partners, with a love that one could reactivate for another partner should one lose this one. For those once-in-a-lifetime situations and predicaments and adventures which require all one's energies to improvise skills, all one's mental powers, all one's emotions and passion are also situations in which one touches at the confines of death. The force of life that finds its identity and its form intact each day for the day's tasks here may be found wanting. They are situations that could only be lived once; the one that expends all his forces on an adventure, that discharges all his mental powers on a problem, that empties out all the love in his heart and sensibility on a woman or a man unlike any other, dies with that adventure, that problem, that love. One senses that; one instinctually arranges one's life so that the tasks and the tools and the problems and the encounters will recur the same each day, one avoids the limits.

Into this succession of days and tasks that recur each day, there come bad hours in which we sense that the forms we have given our lives are coffins. Hours when we can't sleep, and the darkness has blacked out the workplace and the tasks that await us, the costumes and the scenario of the social theater in which we are male or female, the marketplace or the office where we are a salesman or a junior executive. This kind of night can also occur in broad daylight, when the scene and the tracks and the channels seem to disconnect from us. The very recurrence of the days and the day's work gives us the sense that nothing is being accomplished, the kitchen each day has to be cleaned up all over again, the office desk cleared, the assembly line run through again. The paths ahead of one lose their urgency, the way from A to B begins to appear equivalent to that from B to A. The things scattered about no longer support and sustain and demand one. The layout about one loses its relief; it extends bleak and indifferent to one toward featureless horizons. The landscape and its past drift off, the future which the environment marked out in paths that invited one and tasks that summoned one darken over. Emptiness opens up between oneself and the environment, one feels oneself drifting in this void. Anxiety is the sense of the emptiness, the nothingness.

The void that opens up isolates a me that feels itself trembling with anxiety. Anxiety is a premonition of dying, of the phosphorescent environment being extinguished about one, of being cast into nothingness.

Anxiety senses that what death is closing in on is not me, but rather my identity—the form I took on and which was required by tasks and situations, the male or female identity that was demanded by females and males and by jobs and by children. Now this identity seems to have been nothing of my own. Should I die now, the chair in the library before the geometry books will be taken by another student, the punch-press operator I was in the factory will be replaced by another punch-press operator, the sales pitch I had memorized and repeated from client to client will be spoken by another, the male I made myself will be replaced by another body in blue jeans or a business suit, the wife I made myself will be replaced by another body spreading her legs to this man and cooking breakfast in this kitchen for these children. I sense death in my form and identity, nothingness claiming a me that never lived.

What feels anxiety is a heat, a force of life that is potential, not actualized, that clings to itself, and wills to be. When the theater of the practical and social environment fades off into indifference and distance, when the forms my forces have contracted disconnect from the layouts and the functions and the roles, this force of life is backed up against itself, and clings to itself, and feels the cold darkness of nothingness closing in. Isolated, singled out, it feels its own singularity, a force of life assembled in this frail composition of matter, drifting into the abyss, never to be assembled again. This one who had channelled the forces of life into contracting the form of a woman, spouse, mother, hairdresser in a beauty shop, now in the desolate fields of her anxiety feels the inner throbbing of a pulse of life singularly her own, which has never shaped a form of its own, which is imminently threatened with dissolution, and which wills to be.

It is then nothingness that posits being. The blank revelation of nothingness closing in singles out the singular force of a being utterly one's own, on its own. Clinging to itself, feeling itself in the anxiety that pervades its space and moment in the directionless expanses of the darkened universe, this force posits itself, makes its being its own.

Then this singular force and heat of a life one's own finds still, in the drifting dissolution of the instrumental and social environment, a substantial raft of earth under its feet. From the dissolving carpentry of the environment the elemental rises up. This life finds something solid, something supporting, unnameable, that does not crystallize into the recognizable outlines of layouts and well-worn paths that recur across the common and public world of the day. It is once one is backed up into oneself, reduced to the force and will to exist on one's own, that one's groping forces find in the rising up of the elemental unnamed possibilities that answer to oneself alone. A woman finds in her heart a song that is hers alone to sing, that a world has never heard, that if she does not sing it will never be heard. A man finds in the surface and depth of his body the excesses of a passion to love, kisses and caresses to squander upon strangers, upon animals and hills and clouds, such that has never before been felt in the heat of the whirling universe, and if he does not pour forth this passion and this love no organism ever shall, of the countless billions that have come and gone and are on their way.

Out of anxiety, in anxiety, singled out within the unerring arms of death closing in, one finds one's own forces of existing, one finds a compass of elemental possibilities responding to oneself alone, awaiting immemorially for oneself alone.

This finding of being, one's own being, as a power and an exigency that lays claim on one, is conscience.[1] Conscience is first of all an imperative that calls one and orders one to be. The response to this call of one's own being is the fundamental responsibility.

Conscience is not first the order with which the organization of nature and of the practical and social field commands one. Responding to the order and organization of the common world, the layout of the practical and social field is what made one someone, interchangeable with others and replaceable by them. It is what made one make oneself another student, another junior business executive, another lawyer, another husband, another mother, male, female. It is what makes one do, each day, what there is to be done, what makes one say, upon each encounter with another, what one says, what makes one feel, in the midst of each event, what one, what anyone, feels. It is what makes one another one, not on one's own, irresponsible.

One does not hear, and one does not expect to hear, talk about conscience in our classrooms. The profession of professors consists in recycling what has been thought and done and said by others and passing it on to others. One does not find cases of conscience in our public leaders, those media personalities whose elections and executive decrees are determined by human engineering experts who measure the galvanic skin responses of consumers to sound bites and images. One does not find cases of conscience in those who build cities and highways and fill shopping malls and high-rise apartment complexes with wealth. What they produce is determined by the pilot industry of modern capitalism, human engineering, which produces needs and wants in the imaginations of buyers, making them into consumers who consume what others consume.

In our culture it is artists who understand conscience, and understand that it is everything, that without an artist conscience one will only be an entertainer. Someone becomes a singer by saying to himself or herself I have my song to sing, a song that can only come from my voice, my heart, my loneliest loneliness, my unrequited grief, my heart, my nerves and sensibility. This is a power one feels, quivering in all one's organs and glands. It is something one knows by instinct, and which can not be confirmed by teachers, critics, or crowds. The adversary the artist must defeat is not the philistine: what can the tone deaf do to Beethoven? What could the praise, or the criticism, of those who cannot sing mean to Joan Baez? The specific enemy of the artist is the art teacher, whose example tempts one, just for a few hours a day, just to pay the bills, to spend one's time passing on the songs of others to others. Conscience is the sense that I do not have time to take the day off from my music to go on a picnic or the evening off to watch an old favorite on television, do not have the time to pay my bills singing the songs of other to others. The acuteness of conscience is the sting of mortality.

These are the things that Martin Heidegger has seen. The environment into which we are born is already articulated in recurrent and recognizable forms; the formless substance of our forces acquires shape by the words and gestures of others who point out to us the shapes that recur, who show us how to stand and how to eat at tables and how to sit in the places and before the tasks others have vacated, who prompt us to say the things one says and train us to feel the things one feels. Taking the places of others, we make ourselves someone, equivalent to and interchangeable with others.[2] Acquiring the identity of a recurrent and general form, we gear ourselves into the carpentry of the public world, and know the consolation of feeling ourselves each day a pattern on a beginningless, endless tide of functional existence. It is anxiety, the anticipated sense of being cast into nothingness, the death that approaches and singles me out, that singularizes me, that posits my being on its own, that delivers me over to the force of life that is singularly my own.[3] It is the shadow of nothingness approaching that gives me the sense of the end, the end of the life that is singularly my own to live, that disconnects me from the general and recurrent fields of tasks that are for others.[4] The dark shadow of death closing in draws the line of demarcation between the possibilities and tasks that are recurrent, walling them off from me as possibilities and tasks that are for-others, and isolating the range of possibilities and tasks that are for-me.[5] The sense of the end that anxiety contains, the sense of ending, is what assigns an end to every move, and to the whole trajectory of my life. It is what determines ends, ends that are for-me, and an ending for each of my moves. The irreversible direction that my own death assigns to me is what gives direction and directives to each move that is my own.

Heidegger identifies death, identifies it as nothingness. Life, living on one's own, living one's own life, he identifies as determination. To live is to enact determinate movements, not just discharges of the excess forces that a nucleus of life in an organism generates; it is to execute actions, finalized or intentional movements in determined directions, that terminate at objectives. It is to build a dwelling, to care for living things and to maintain monuments of immortal things.[6] Heidegger has taken up the Spinozist formulation that *omnis determinatio est negatio*: every determination is a line fixed between what is and what is not, between what a being is and how far it goes, and from there on not-that-being, nothing. It is nothingness that delimits, determines, being. Then, to posit being is to encounter nothingness. Ex-istence, the movement of force by which a being casts itself out of its present here-and-now position, is experience. The most negative experience, the anticipated casting oneself, with all one's own forces, into nothingness itself, is also the most positive, positing, experience, the movement that posits one's being on its own, that makes one exist on one's own, that makes the force of life in one one's own.

This Heideggerian vision, when embraced, when lived, reveals, it seems to us, the following obscurities.

Is it really possible that dying, ending, is what gives direction and directive to our life? The oncoming of death, according to Heidegger, is what circumscribes, in the general field of possibilities that are possibilities for-anyone, the definite and determinate range of possibilities that are for-me. Death is to-come, it is the very region of futurity, and the anticipated projection of my powers over the range of possibilities open about me all the way to the end is what reveals the future that is open singularly to me. Anxiety, which is the premonition of the nothingness to come, is the movement in every anticipation and every projection, is the sense of the possible in every anticipation and in every fear. The apprehensiveness before the oncoming of nothingness is in every apprehension that grasps hold of the beings at hand.

But can death really function in this way? For death, which is certainly my future, is not in the future; it does not lie ahead of the field of possibilities open before me. Death is imminent at every moment; it is not a moment that lies ahead of the succession of moments before me, it is an event immanent in every event. The last moment may be the next moment. The contingency of the being that is promised in the moment is its possible impossibility. Death is everywhere in the environment; every step I take may plunge me into the abyss, every objective that offers itself to my reach may be the ambush from which there will be no advance and no return. The location and the approach of death cannot be surveyed across the line and distance of the future; anxiety feels it cold up against me, latent in the apparent tranquillity and assurance of the things at hand. Death which has no front lines cannot be confronted. It cannot fix a direction; the groping hand of life touches it everywhere, just beneath the apparent support of all surfaces that rest and that phosphoresce in their places.

Heidegger began by radically separating the observation of the dying of others from the inner certainty I have of being mortal. The observation of the dying of others, he wrote, observes the transformation of the self-moving organism of another into the rest and immobility of a corpse, which is essentially tranquillizing: nothing perceptible has been annihilated; the spectacle of being is as full as before. But my own sense of being mortal is anxiety; it is the sense of the possibility of the whole spectacle of reality about me dissolving into void and of the onward and irreversible thrust of my own being into nothingness. But, later in his book, he says that death, nothingness, which has no dimensions, cannot fix a line of direction and impose a directive.[7] It is, he writes, from the dying of others that I find inscribed on the world the direction and the directive that will actualize the forces that are my own. For everyone who sets out to blaze forth his own path with the powers that are singularly his own also sketches out other paths that are also open singularly to him. Each one who sets out to actualize the dancer, thinker, lover he alone can be also catches sight of the painter, poet, man of action he also alone has the power to be. In resolutely setting out to realize the thinker she was born to be, she sketches out, and leaves for others, the dancer, lover, mystic she also was born to be. He and she leave these paths traced out in the world, and I who come upon them find on them the directives for a life singularly my own.

Heidegger identifies death. He identifies death with nothingness, dying with the passing from existing to nothingness. But this identification seems to us fraught with obscurities. Does it not belong to the essence of death that it is radically ungraspable, inapprehendable, uncomprehendable? It is not only the moment and place of death that is unlocatable; it is that death, which is imminent in every moment and in every site, has no identity. Although it is certain that each of us is singled out by death, what it is that closes in upon us and singles us out is the unknown. Death is not the line over which we look to identify being and nothingness; it is the line between the determinable and the indeterminable. What we do know is that once we cross this line there will be no return. Death is the interminable. It is too much to try to say to assert that we can identify that which has no identity, as nothingness. The act of identification seeks to apprehend something one and the same in the unutterably singular, singularizing death that closes in on each one. Each one dies with his own death; it is in the place singled out by death that each one of us is not equivalent to and interchangeable with another.

It is true that sometimes we know the proximity of the end. Its close presence is held in the focus of our will, is seen in the bottle of sleeping pills within our reach, in the alien will of another visible in his hostile eyes and revolver bracketed on us, in the inexorable progression of the cancer. Indeed we sense it within in every illness, in every pain, in every fatigue and weariness. But between the last moment, absolute cut in the line of time, and now, there extends the time of dying. Death, the absolutely other, inapprehendable, unlocatable, advances, of itself. But in the space of time before the end, one is held in the time of dying—a time in which death is at work before it strikes, effacing already all possibilities. One finds oneself adrift in a now that prolongs itself, disconnected from the time of projects and tasks and possibilities, disconnected from the time and the tasks of the others who come to keep one company in this immobile, immobilizing movement. One finds oneself in a time that is without possibilities— there is nothing one can do to elude the advance of death, nothing one can do to propel the thrust of life. The now does not give way to the future, that is, to tasks and possibilities. The past is likewise disconnected; it is retained, recaptured, represented in the thrust of life that propels itself into possibilities and tasks with the momentum and the direction of the past. Now, in the time of dying, the lessons and the force of the past drift off into inefficacity and insignificance. The present pulse of life no longer gathers up what has come to pass in it to direct itself into what awaits it ahead. Coming from nowhere, going nowhere, drifting, the now prolongs itself without force or sense. There is nothing to do but suffer. This suffering endures its prostration, undergoes its prostrate endurance. There is nothing to understand, for anything or for anyone. What closes in on one concerns oneself alone. Unable to parry and unable to flee and unable to retreat, life finds itself mired in itself—not in a self that stands by itself and holds itself together—but in a self depersonalized that is reduced of function, role, form, identity, that does not take hold of its death but is taken in advance by death. Dying is this suffering, this transubstantiation from activity to passivity and prostration, this materialization. One dies from a world, one dies into a world.

In this passage not from being into nothingness but from activity to passivity that comes to pass in illness, in pain, in fatigue and weariness, there is nonetheless an understanding and an accompaniment. For there is understanding in undergoing suffering. One suffers as one suffers, as anyone, everything that lives suffers, as all flesh suffers. In the endurance and the patience of this passivity, one draws near to everyone that suffers and that dies, to the famished and the tortured and the massacred, to the great elephants that die in the swamps and the sparrows that die in the cold, to the butterflies that die in the sun and the burrowing animals that die in the dark of the earth, to the lonely stars that die in the voids of universe, to the Assyrian and African gods that die as the deserts grow and the Maya gods that die as the rain forests burn.

Socrates, father of philosophy, claimed to know nothing, claimed no intellectual powers or pedagogical virtues; instead, at his trial he reminded his accusers of three occasions that they all knew in which he had shown his courage. Aristotle placed courage first in the list of virtues; it is not only first of the list of virtues, but the transcendental virtue, the virtue that makes the other virtues possible, for neither magnanimity nor friendship nor piety nor truthfulness nor even wit in conversation are possible without courage.[8] Heidegger believed he was following Socrates and Aristotle by making of the resolute confrontation of death the power, the virtue, that makes authenticity possible. But there is perhaps a still greater courage in the one who comes to accompany the other in his or her dying, the one who comes not to visit and help the sick one in the hospital but to stay when there is no longer anything to do and no help or consolation is possible, the one who comes to stay with the dying one until the end comes. The hand extended to the dying one communicates no information and brings no relief and knows no hope, is there only to accompany the other in his or her dying, to suffer and to die with him or her. And in this hand there is perhaps an understanding more profound than all apprehension and all comprehension, a force stronger than every efficacity and a compassion beyond and beneath every virtue—the hand extended to the starved child in Ethiopia and Calcutta, the hand extended to the butterfly dying in the sun.

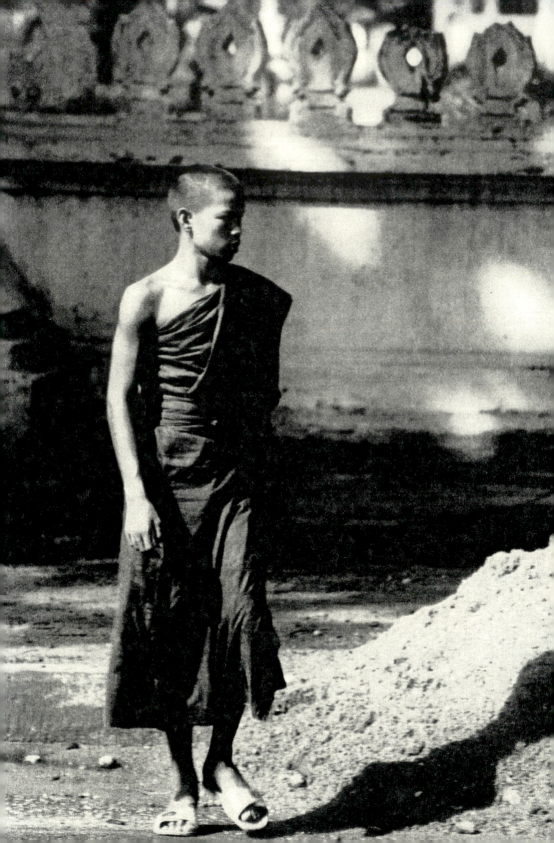

2

◆

The World as a Whole

Martin Heidegger's *Being and Time*[1] set out to show that understanding, feeling, and action are elements of a structural whole. Affectivity, action, and understanding are integrated temporally, Heidegger explains, as the past, present, and future dimensions of one temporal trajectory. But this structural whole only exists within a relationship with the environment—with the whole environment. For, Heidegger claims, what we understand, feel, and act upon is the world.

There are two different ways that *Being and Time* shows that our experience is not simply an experience of our perceived environment, an *Umwelt*, or of the immanent organization of our sensations, but of the world. On the one hand, Heidegger shows that our moves outward, which are simultaneously perceptual, affective, and practical—movements of concern—reach out for implements and obstacles in a practicable layout, whose instrumental connections extend on indefinitely. Here "the world" is the distribution, the layout as such; it is the teleological finality, the ordinance, that makes the multiplicity of beings about us an order, a cosmos. It is the open-ended network of instrumental connections.

On the other hand, the world is given in moods. In moods, the whole figures as that which weighs on us, that to which we are subjected. Practical activity may weary, and lose interest in the practicable world. Boredom disconnects us from the tasks at hand, and drifts over a landscape where nothing lures, nothing promises, where all paths sink into equivalence. But the environment oppresses us by its very desolation. At the limit of boredom, nothingness itself shows through this generalized insignificance. Anxiety feels the oppressive weight of the abysses of nothingness and death. In this nothingness the world appears in its contingency and as a whole. But it makes itself felt as an unarticulated and oppressive density and a burden.

The practicable field comprehensively grasped as an open-ended instrumental complex and the massive and unarticulated whole pressing down immediately

13

upon us with all its weight in mood are in discord. Does Heidegger succeed in showing that these two guises of totality are the future and past dimensions of a movement by which the world presents itself at each moment of experience? Or, will we find that the world comes apart in this discord?

THE FORM OF THE WORLD

Being and Time elaborates an antisubstantive ontology not only of our existence, but also of intramundane things. Things[2] are described not as substances but as relays of force, grasped on the move, as we reach for them and manipulate them. They are means and intermediaries. They are made to appear so by the Heideggerian analysis which emphasizes their forms rather than their materiality: their composition or their sensuous opacity and the inertia of their resistance.[3] These forms are not simply shapes, boundaries, contours; they are dynamic axes, concretizations of orientation. The features we catch sight of in things are not properties but modes of appropriateness. To encounter something in our practicable environment is to grasp the serviceable and reliable, or run up against the recalcitrant and detrimental. The understanding that identifies things is not a contemplating what is here in front of one now; it is a touching upon what is here as a relay on the way to what this thing is oriented toward, what it leads to, what it conducts one to. To go to the cellar and find a hammer is to spot something that can serve to pound in the nail or crack the walnuts. To recognize a vertical plane as a door is to see that one can open it and exit through it; to see a horizontal plane as a corridor is to see it as capable of sustaining our movement across it. To see something is to see what it is for; we see not shapes but possibilities.

We produce the logically possible by taking what is present contingently before us, through perception, and representing it, by imagination, in other arrangements. Something is really possible, however, only if the alternative position in which one imagines it is possibly impossible. To see that one can bicycle to Pittsburgh is to foresee that one's tires may blow, one's gears break. Nothing useful is useful only for an instant, nor forever; all things, in being used, are used up.[4] Recalcitrance, wear, possible breakdown are constitutive of the serviceability and reliability of implements. What understands that it is possible to pound in the tack or the spike with this hammer is not a logical intellect that represents alternative positions of terms identified, but our practical power to grasp hold of the hammer and manipulate it. Sensing the recalcitrance of things, our hand senses its possible impotence.

Relays of force, the things surface in a field of possibilities, an instrumental field. The instrumental complex makes possible the emergence and the form of an implement. We opened doors and saw at a glance that this is the kitchen, this the bathroom, this the bedroom. In the one setting a bottle of amber oil emerges as possibly cooking oil, in another as possibly soap, in another as possibly genital lubricant.

Every end is a possible means for further ends; the instrumental connections of any field in which we act extend indefinitely. Heidegger concludes that the practical environment does not consist of a succession of fragmentary and discontinuous fields, but is, from the first and always, *the world*.

The instrumental connections that extend from hammer to nails to shingles to house sheltering the implements of life from the inclemencies of the weather end up at the agent who will inhabit that house (or another house, for the acquisition of which building this house will be the means). It is in conceiving a possible position for himself in the midst of things, and plunging toward that future position, that an agent extends the great arc in which the world takes form, a world in which all things are means and intermediaries.

There is a comprehension of the layout of the world ahead in the every movement of the hand. The stance and momentum of an agent retains the orientation and lines of force of the field behind him. The agent who is fully engaged in his action integrates the temporal trajectory of his life from his birth to his death in each of his projects.

If nothing useful is useful for an instant only, no implement is only a correlate of the momentary diagram of the move of my hand. An implement is open to a range of manipulations, and the hand that hammers strikes the nail with equivalent and interchangeable blows. The agent sees others acting with movements equivalent to and interchangeable with his own. The field in which one acts is from the first open to anyone. An agent begins to act by picking up diagrams of movement from others; the common world precedes and makes possible the practicable environment of any individual. A practical movement one sees another making is an interpretation: the shallow dish at the formal dinner is a finger-bowl; the vinyl-covered bench is for body massage. The interpretative system of gestures, and the language, picked up from others, passed on to others, precedes and makes possible any singularizing interpretation of one's own situation.

THE WORLD BROKEN UP BY ACTION

The hand that grips the hammer and manipulates it forms a functional unit with it. As the size and weight of the board calls for nails of a certain length and strength, and the gauge of the nails calls for a certain hammer, the weight and balance of the hammer calls for a certain grip of the hand and swing and force of the arm. The implements induce us to assess ourselves in instrumental terms. This everyday practical motivation is so strong that, Heidegger says,

virtually all science and philosophy understand the human agent with the categories and relations that hold for things materialized within the world. The
apprehension of any tool presupposes a comprehensive survey of the layout of
the world, but then the layout fades out and leaves only the functional unit of
hand, hammer, nails, and shingles.

An agent who forms his forces according to diagrams read off from the
implements fits himself into a series of equivalent and interchangeable agents.
One takes the place another has vacated before the punch press and makes the
operations with the rhythm the punch press dictates, making oneself another
punch press operator. One opens the geometry text and recycles the demon-
strations of Euclid in one's cerebral circuitry, making oneself another student.
One experiences oneself as a figure on a wave of operations picked up from
others, passed on to others. One makes oneself *uneigentlich*, not existing and
acting "on one's own." The world disintegrates into discontinuous functional
units, but the agent experiences himself as continuous with other agents.

The apprehension of oneself as part of an instrumental system is not simply
the result of the incompossibility of viewing the whole world and also viewing
functional entities in their clarity and distinctness—the inevitable "erring" that
produces error.[5] The agent clings to the things at hand; there is fear in his
concern. He shrinks back from the open horizons. The open paths and horizons of the layout are open with, suspended in, the abyss of nothingness, of
which he has a premonition in anxiety. The cognitive conflict between the
holistic comprehension of the world and the reifying view of oneself as a set of
operations on the implements at hand owes its force to the opposition between anxiety and fear.

The actual that presents the diagram of the really possible is inwardly hol-
lowed out by the possibility of impossibility. To be concerned about things, to
care for them, is not only to cherish them but also to worry about them. The
apprehension of the possible involves apprehensiveness before the impossible.
The sense of the impossible as such, given in the anxiety which senses the
nothingness in which the layout of the contingent world is suspended and into
which it is destined, precedes and makes possible the sense of possibilities in
the things at hand. The preoccupation with things moves with the force of
anxiety.

The actual, which materializes a concrete figure of possibility, holds the eyes
and the hand, and breaks the vertiginous premonition of the abyss. One clings
to the things within reach, one fits oneself into them. One holds one's eyes
fixed on the possible figure of one's force that will materialize in them in order
to flee the inner sense of the movement in one's being that casts one into the
layout of the world and the void in which it is mapped. The things are rafts

and refuges which we cling to in fleeing the uncanny sense of nothingness that the sense of openness opens upon.

The agent does not sweep his workshop or repair his truck as one maintaining the machinery of the world, but as one of a team anxiously keeping afloat a life-raft in the dark abysses of nothingness. Heidegger argues that since the preoccupation with the things at hand is only possible as a fear of the open horizons beyond, the experience of the world as a whole precedes and makes possible the practical concern with one's immediate environment. But his argument shows that what makes the open horizons fearful is not their world-structure—the continuity of instrumental connections in all directions—but the radical discontinuity, the abyss, that paralyzes anxiety.

A SITUATION OF ONE'S OWN

In conceiving a future position for himself the agent extends a world in which all things are means and intermediaries, but that future position is not a stable and final state. It is only possible, that is, possibly impossible. Death is everywhere in the world; a path may lead to an ambush, a step fall into a snare, an implement may splinter, shatter, electrocute, or poison the water or the air. The future impossibility of one's position is a real and not only conceptual impossibility; one's position is possibly impossible because it is eventually impossible. Anxiety is the premonition of the final and total impossibility. The future state of the agent for whom all means and all mundane ends are means is its nonexistence.

Yet it is the sense of the possible impossibility in the things at hand that also brings to flush their real possibilities. Death, which terminates my powers, determines and makes determinate the real possibilities in things ahead of me. These are the possibilities that answer to the powers that are singularly one's own—*eigentlich*, one's authentic powers. The agent finds himself having to contrive actions of his own before tasks singularly his own, which will pass as the singular situation passes. The real paths and implements he finds do not offer him possibilities to rest and endure supported by them, but possibilities to move on in an itinerary that is destined for the end. The resoluteness *Being and Time* propounds would manipulate and use things as means not to materialize one's future position in the layout of the world, but to relay one's trajectory toward the abyss. Action would be discharging one's forces into things, dying in them. Action dies away in order that the world become determinate.

The agent who is fully engaged in his action integrates the temporal trajectory of his life from his birth to his death in each of his projects. While the range of possibilities within reach in the environment about him are delimited and determined by the death he anticipates, they, relays offered his itinerary, are unilaterally integrated; they form the unity of his "situation." Once one recognizes the scope of possibilities really possible for oneself, one comes to recognize the distinctiveness of the situation in which each of the others act. Yet the singularity of one's own situation and the distinctiveness of those of others appear as ways about which are each time organized differently the possibilities possible for anyone which make up the common world.

Thus the agent who anticipates his end and takes hold of the powers that are singularly his own experiences his discontinuity from all other agents, but experiences the continuity of the common world from which his own discontinuous situation arises in relief.

What, then, is new in Heidegger is not only positing a real experience of the world as a whole, but locating this experience in an agent become discontinuous and singular. But crucial moves in Heidegger's reasoning seem to us unintelligible. And his phenomenological description of authentic action seems to us skewed.

Heidegger argues that the sense of the irreversible propulsion of a life toward its end precedes and makes possible every unilateral array of means toward particular ends and every determinate action. But can death, which has no front lines and no dimensions, assign a determinate direction to one's life, and thereby impart a unilateral direction to the connections in the instrumental field? The anxiety that anticipates dying does not anticipate a last moment situated in the time of the world which my existence extends. Death is neither present nor future; it is imminent at any moment. How could death then fix the end and bring to flush the ends possible in the time that lies ahead?

Heidegger concedes that the path of one's own destiny, which unifies one's life and one's situation, cannot be drawn from the nothingness of death.[6] He then argues that it is in the common world, in paths inscribed on the world by others, that one finds the possibilities left for one and for which one's own powers are destined. Yet he would have to explain that the lives of others trace out paths of possibility which they leave for others because the path they actualized was an assignation put on them by death. The explanation only displaces the question.

In Heidegger's dialectic, anxiety, the most negative experience, experience of nothingness itself, converts into the most positive experience, positing my existence as my own, positing the world in its totality. The entry into the world as my home passes through the most extreme degree of alienation. Out of an experience of the actuality on hand and of the impossibility that infiltrates into it from the abyss, the world emerges as a field of possibility. Is there not an insurmountable unintelligibility at the core of this account, where the world is identified both as being and as nonbeing, its contents identified as possibilities made of actuality and impossibility? To the dialectic that seeks to retrace the genesis of the world, Maurice Merleau-Ponty objected that distance, differentiation, gradation, pregnancy are primitive notions and that the facticity and nothingness with which dialectics constructs them are twin abstractions.[7]

Anxiety functions ambiguously in Heidegger as the abstraction that yields an experience of nothingness but also that disengages the preoccupation with what is at hand so as to survey being in its totality. The experience of pure nothingness would not be an experience; the Heideggerian anxiety, like the Cartesian doubt or the Husserlian imaginative annihilation of the world, posits one's own being and, unlike the Cartesian doubt or the Husserlian imaginative annihilation of the world, stations it resolutely upon its own mundane situation. Nothingness then becomes the factor of discrimination and differentiation internal to the extension of the world. How could nothingness, which has no front lines and no dimensions, which is not between moments of presence but imminent in them, function to differentiate and to defer?

The ambiguity persists in Heidegger's later writings where our home in the world is laid out upon the supporting substance of the earth but also under open skies, extended by the harbingers of the holy but also by the morality that is in our own essence. Death then is not the permanent and imminent threat that gapes open about our inhabitation in the world, but is a constitutive element of that inhabitation. Yet Heidegger continues to speak of the world harbored in the "shrine of nothingness."[8]

DISCONTINUOUS EPOCHS, DISCONTINUOUS SITUATIONS

The shingles, the roof, the house, the climate in Freiburg, the winds that come over the Alps are connected when the carpenter reaches for the hammer—but are Pennsylvania, Madagascar, the black holes of the Andromeda Galaxy, Auschwitz, the gods of the Yanomamö also? They will be located progressively by researchers in geography, geology, astronomy, by military espionage, and by anthropological fieldwork. The world is a progressive, temporal synthesis, or transitional synopsis, Merleau-Ponty says.

The authentic life that integrates its temporal trajectory from its birth to its death in each of its projects finds its own possibility traced out, Heidegger explains in *Being and Time*,[9] and left for it by those who pursued their own paths to their own deaths. The hero finds his own destiny in the unfulfilled tasks left by heroes before him; a thinker finds his own task in what was foreseen but not elaborated by thinkers before him; a farmer finds his own life's work in the plans and also integrity of the life of his father. Thus the one who finds in the world his own task makes the whole of what has come to pass not be bygone. As *Being and Time* teaches that the instrumental connections that organize one's own sphere of operations extend continuously across the common world, so it teaches that each one, taking up the possibilities traced out by those who lived authentically before him, makes the world common and continuous across time.

But in his later writings, Heidegger shows that the time of the world breaks into discontinuous epochs, without causal determination or dialectical implication discoverable among them, without a logic of history. The world loses its continuity, at least in its duration.

Is that not also true of the environment of any individual? Does it not happen that we find the onward drift of our environment disconnected from our actual movements and operations? Does not each life extend across metamorphoses, in which it finds itself reborn with tasks that were nowhere yesterday; does it not find whole fragments of its past drifting behind it, unintegratable like dreams in the daylight reality about it?

We go to the cellar to fix a broken chair with drill, screws, and glue; the phone rings and we plan a trip with a friend, mapping out an itinerary, jotting down things that have to get done—have the car greased and oiled, get a passport, arrange for injections from the doctor; suddenly there is a scream and we drop the phone, hurtle out the door and grab a stick to thrash the cat that has caught a blue jay; on the way back to the house we glance at our watch and realize it is almost time for our appointment with the hypnotist to stop smoking . . .

The one that grasps the hammer does not comprehensively envision the carpentry of the whole world. The practicable fields are limited and discontinuous. Between and beyond them, there are innumerable impracticable fields. Does anyone inhabit the universe?

Heidegger later came to see things not as crystallizing in the axes of a field of instrumental paths already there, but as locations which extend places and foci which assemble the dimensions for the world. In the late essay "The Thing," he contrasts the et cetera of objects generated by the formulas of technological production[10] with the few and inconspicuous things[11] where we are brought into the presence of the axes of earth and skies, mortals and the harbingers of the sacred—the world. The priority of the world with regard to any implement that takes form, put forth in *Being and Time*, is reversed; it is in the proximity with things that the most remote axes of the world become present.

But do not the horizons close in, the beckoning paths fade out, the gearings and the axes of force thicken and become opaque when we come to dwell in things? About the few things that are really things with which we live—an old coffee mug, a carved and padded armchair, a violin, a pearl-oyster shell on the window sill—does not the wide world, the common world, break up into so many discontinuous spaces full of dreams and memories? Even more, do not these spaces themselves etiolate and get absorbed into the opaque substance of those things, like the root of the chestnut tree before Roquentin thickening into something unnameable in any world?

Heidegger's analysis, axed not on the material but on the forms a practical life manipulates in the dynamic field, argues that things are essentially means; each mundane end is a means in turn. The relay from implement to implement and to work being done returns to the manipulator. Before the hand grasps the hammer, this whole circuit must have already been laid out. The handling is a movement that fits in this comprehensive system and is determined by it from the start.

But does not the finality in things also come to an end in them? Water which one knows in the savoring and in the drinking, berries which one gathers and which melt in one's mouth as one walks through the meadow do not catch our eye as refurbishments for our cells and muscles and means for our projects; they are substances in which sensuality glows and fades away. The materiality of things is not just there as the materialization of the dynamic form we grasp; once grasped and brought under one's eyes and in one's home, the instrumental forms of things dissolve into the density of their substance. The movement of the carpenter that takes hold of the hammer passes through it to the nails and the shingles and the house and the stormy skies and the work done in the home to be sheltered. But once on the job, this relay-course of finalities dissolves into sunlight and bracing air, and in his hand his hammer becomes a rhythm that prolongs itself. He can be contented with that, contented with hammering in the sun.[12] The objective intention thickens into a sensual attention that ends in the hammer, and the carpenter can enjoy the rhythm and reverberation of the hammering and enjoy this very activity as a content. One walks down the path to get somewhere, but one enjoys walking, and one can leave one's house just to walk. Is it really true that the vision that sweeps over the landscape sees so much resources, tools, a cosmic machinery? One sees the fields rippling with the meaningless hum of insects, the rhythmic flow of the green hills, the sky speckled with birds veering and reversing. Does not the carpenter whose hammering goes smoothly, by itself—a rhythm that prolongs itself of itself rather than an operation being piloted by an intentionality—whose eyes drift over the landscape and the street below, lose himself in patterns and contours of substance?

The movement of the hand does not have the technical efficiency of a movement lined up to an instrumental layout already laid out. There is not first a project, a plan, a finality before the hand activates; it reaches out, grasps, tears up, kneads, crushes. There is an element of groping, Emmanuel Levinas says,[13] in the most skilled manipulations. As one works at one's workbench in the cellar, building a cabinet, the layout fades back continually into the indeterminate; one fumbles for the hammer, the screw driver, the screw one just put down and which have already sunk into the sensuous density of the environment.

Heidegger sees especially in the handling of implements the basic comprehensive movement, which understands their identities and their functions; the hand moves as a sense organ, gathering information. But it moves also as a sensuous organ, fondling substances and textures, fondling the silk and the velvet and the moss and the downy hands of a lover, rubbing out the shapes of things to reduce them to buoyant or fluid or vaporous depth or solidity that extends indefinitely into the depths of the earth. It enjoys the random play of its movements, enjoys being surprised.

The hand that reaches out for things does not make the outside more and more determinate. As one works, as the cabinet takes form under one's hands, the working space fills up with wood shavings, tools left here and there in disarray, spilled nails. One makes one's way down the paths of the garden to look for the onions for one's meal or to gather flowers for a bouquet, and one leaves, and leaves the rest to rest or to drift in the indeterminate. As one makes a meal, the kitchen space fills up with knives and mixing bowls, husks and scrapings, and pots and pans in disorder. Action then does not lay out the axes and determinations and instrumental connections of the world. It stakes out a zone of the practicable, and in inhabiting it, this zone transforms or unforms into an unpracticable density in which one rests and dreams. Heidegger's concept of the *Vorhanden*, the stock of forms on hand which lends itself to the measurement and calculation of objectifying representation, does not capture the substantiality into which the forms of instrumentality subside, and which not the intentions but the sensuality of the body recognizes. Beyond the alignment of implements in the great arc of the practicable world which closes back upon the agent, this substantiality extends in fathomless depth.

THE WEIGHT OF THE WORLD

We cannot survey our environment without being concerned with it. As soon as we open our eyes, the room, the landscape opening from our window, and the skies above beset us, soliciting, enticing, badgering. The exterior is not an empty and neutral, but a resplendent and laughing or desolate and oppressive space. The environment, whose forms our practical look surveys, is felt to affect us, weighs on us; its materiality matters to us.

Heidegger distinguishes between emotion and mood. An emotion is a movement outward upon an objective perceived as alluring or threatening. Moods are ways we are tuned in to the whole layout, or ways the layout reverberates and resonates in us. The emotion of fear arises on the ground of a mood of disquietude and vulnerability. It is because one senses oneself from the first subjected to indifferent or inimical reality that emotion is not a view held on an object from a distance, but is held by it and specifically affective.

Moods are pervasive; they are for Heidegger the second way the world is there as a whole. The world is grasped formally in the practical looking about and looking for and is sensed materially in mood.

Feeling is a contact-sense; mood is the sense of the world in its density and opacity. The arid spread of the roads and the bleak hills, the oppressive darkness of the skies above are not just viewed at a distance; we feel, within ourselves, their oppressive weight. In uneasiness and in dread, our eyes scan the environs, it seems to us that the surfaces of things, like blind masks, harbor dangers and threats; the menacing substance of nearby and remote things weighs heavy against us, and we feel it in the coldness of our skin and the unsteadiness of our nerves and legs.

In and through feeling, things, and the world, are *given*. For being to be given is not just to be deposited there, in front of us. What really is, what is given, is not just a pattern hovering before our eyes, and which may be a will-o'-the-wisp, an image, a memory, or a dream. What is given crowds in on us, imposes itself on us, weighs on us. For us to find ourselves (*sich befinden*) is to find ourselves as subjects, and this does not mean as spontaneous or creative source-points; it means as loci of subjection.

We stand on the top of the mountain and view Qosqo below us, and if it does not seem to us that simply there are so many lines extending across the field of our vision, as when we stand in front of a map or a painting, it is because we feel the distance, the vastness of the space. Our eyes do not only delineate the serpentine crawl of the road, the core of the old colonial city and the recent shantytowns about it, the ancient Indian hamlets in the hills, and the strata and fault lines of the Andes under the vacant skies, but we feel the enormity of historical and geological and cosmic time compressing the brief thrust of our lifetime.

Tedium, the sense that nothing matters, that all the things spread out in town for us to occupy ourselves with are tawdry and pointless, is a suffering, a suffocating; in the inconsequentiality of the tasks we feel oppressed by the world that afflicts us with those tasks. On vacation, at first we feel elated to be freed from our post before a layout of tasks and obligations, full of things we have to do every waking hour. We find ourselves at a resort where the maids bring our meals, do our laundry, clean the sink after us, make the bed, the waiters bring our meals. Now it is the very emptiness of a practical field where all the resistances and obstacles have been removed that weighs on us, and after two weeks of this we feel weary and exhausted with the weight of the days, we find it harder and harder to move under the vacancy of vacation. Indolence is a suffering; one has to endure the weight of the emptiness where there is nothing to do. People who are rich and have nothing they have to do, and who rush about to entertainments and pastimes are fleeing the weight of the emptiness of the days and of the world.[14]

Heidegger emphasizes this sense of burden there is in the given; the world weighs on us, we cannot be indifferent to it, cannot elude it; we cannot just focus in on some implement or some curiosity and ignore the pressure of the being in which we are submerged. When Heidegger later speaks, with Rilke, of the environment that "opens up" about us, the *Lichtung*, he takes pains to explain that a zone of radiance and light opens because the density and weight of things has been thinned out, as in a forest clearing full of light where the things can be luminously seen because the thickness of the forest has been cleared away. It seems odd to speak of the world felt first as a weight and as burdensome when we are in a mood of elation or exhilaration—but, Heidegger says, elation, the sense of the lightness of being, the sense of buoyancy and bounding force, is the sense of alleviation of the burden of being and thus presupposes and reveals it.[15] Here is another of the places where his thinking is dialectical: one cannot feel buoyancy and lightness except in contrast with the heaviness and turgidity also felt, and indeed felt more deeply beneath all elation. Why not say that the oppressive, burdensome sense of the world presupposes the more basic sense of the lightness of the clearing about us? But even the sense of the world being light, floating, inconsistent is an affliction; Milan Kundera wrote of the unbearable lightness of being.

Every mood, boredom or exhilaration, anxiety or serenity, throws one up against the blank, contingent fact of one's being there, of having been cast there. "Mood brings Dasein before the 'that-it-is' of its 'there,' which, as such, stares it in the face with the inexorability of an enigma," Heidegger writes.[16] Every mood is a bewilderment. "Even if Dasein is 'assured' in its belief about its 'whither,' or if, in rational enlightenment, it supposes itself to know about its 'whence,' all this counts for nothing"[17] as against the enigmatic and bare fact of being there at all. The massive presence of the world closes off its past and its future.

As one throws oneself into one's initiatives and projects, one finds oneself already here in some contingent spot, implanted in a here in the density of actuality. This is not something that one observes, as one locates facts in predrawn coordinates; it is something one feels—by, Heidegger says, turning away from it. It is by looking up the road and toward the horizon that one senses that one is here as a matter of fact.

By uneasily turning from what is in front of one, looking for destinations, envisioning a layout of paths and possibilities, one seeks to elude the massive presence not of some thing that may obstruct one's path, but of the world itself weighing down upon one. One flees the weight of the world into the extension of the world; one flees the materiality of the world into its form.

The evasion is the first movement, the inner diagram of every movement. It is by turning away from the locus where one is, subjected to the weight of the world, that one envisions the open-ended layout of instrumental connections that is the form of the world. Then, the form of the world does not inform its materiality; they are separated as the future and past of a present movement which is evasion.

Moreover, it seems that the sense of subjection does not totalize the density of the environment, and the initiative does not totalize the layout into the form of the world. If the initiative of evasion is possible, it is because the mood feels itself weighted down with a district, or a surge, of reality (with indistinct limits), and not the totality. If the initiative declares that the open-ended layout of a practicable field is a zone where the oppressive weight of reality can be evaded, this layout does not extend to the ends of the world. For the materiality of reality felt in mood obturates our view, weighs down our hands and our eyes with weariness such that we are embedded in the density that settles down upon us and see very little.

Yet Heidegger says that through the sense of weight felt immediately on the here where we find ourselves, the totality is sensed. On the shoulders of the one whose eyes seek out another position in the clearing ahead, the enormity of material reality presses. The tedium that loosens one's grip on one's implements feels not their resistance circumscribed within contours, but the unending recurrence of days beyond the day's work, the dust of the world beyond the dirt on the floor. For Heidegger it is the pressure of nothingness that lays the weight of the whole environment upon each of us from the start. It is also the pressure of nothingness that makes the form of the world inform the materiality of the world, that slips the future over the past.

Heidegger follows the movement that carries action into boredom and into anxiety. The effective action that reads off its directives from the materials it acts on and from its implements and from the diagrams of action of other agents acting on equivalent materials and with equivalent implements discovers itself to be an operation that recurs or can recur every day and in any place. Where the trajectory of the day returns the following day as though nothing is attained, the path from A to B appears equivalent to that from B to A; nothing lures, nothing promises, and boredom senses the environment that oppresses by its very desolation. The dissolution of the imperatives in tasks and implements and of the weight of obstacles into a generalized insignificance and indifference gives way to the weight of the void itself. The pressure of the void breaks down our purposive stances before tasks at hand into the staggerings of anxiety. Anxiety is equivocally the sense of the massive weight of the totality and the sense of the void behind and in the weight of the world.

In Heidegger's account, for the hand that reaches out for an implement the layout of instrumental connections extends without end, suspended over the void. For feeling, the exterior presses down upon it, as an unarticulated weight, whether that exterior is felt to be the weight of being or of the void. How are these two different guises of the exterior identified as the world? Through the intermediary of nothingness: if want, lack, deficiency, or shortfall determine the contours that contain a particular entity, nothingness itself would totalize all being—that extended before us as an instrumental layout and that weighing massively on us in mood—as the world.

Yet it is not an external but an internal factor that could make what is contained within contours an individual and what is excluded from nothingness a whole. The open-ended field of action gets its unity from the dynamic continuity of its instrumental connections. The nothingness over which it is extended threatens it at every point. The sense of nothingness besetting the environment that is felt pressing down on one would not make that environment so much a whole or a world as a bounded exteriority.

We asked above whether the paradoxical ontology that works with the concept of a real possibility made of actuality and impossibility, with the concepts of being and nothingness, is not ultimately unintelligible. We think it is phenomenologically unfaithful. We think that what there is is not the world extended in the abysses which anxiety divines. We think there are multiple and discontinuous practicable and impracticable fields, extended not in the void but in the sensuous density.

The eyes open and are flooded by the light. The gaze that extends is buoyed up by the radiance. The posture that forms, the feet that advance, and the hand that gropes do so in the density of the support that extends a ground and rises in outcroppings and in things resting in their stations. The voice that murmurs takes up the currents of the air and sends its vibration into them.

A field of paths and obstacles opens in the light. The light itself is not a network of instrumental references but a sensuous medium. Contours of the graspable surface in the density of the night. Signals and threats take form in the rumble of the city, in the murmurs of nature. These are not maps extending in the void. A traffic sign solidifies in the flow of the landscape and of the radiations of the night. Clouds shift in the blue radiance of the sky. Stars beam in the hard density of the night. Our desk takes form in the generalized chromatic tone of a room which is not a spaceship in uncharted voids but a harbor in the warm and perfumed density of the resounding night. The jug glows not in the intersection of axes it extends but in the tranquillity of the home.

The light does not open about us like an epiphany of possibilities upon possibilities; its very radiance fills and thickens the space such that the surfaces of gleaming or dark things at a distance are dissolved in it. The rumble of the city, the murmur of nature, the din of the night does not extend about us as so many potential sounds accessible to our discernment; the hubbub of a party makes it impossible to hear even the one standing in front of us. The mossy bark our hand touches in the density of the night holds our movement and does not release it for the rest which is sunken into obscurity.

The light, the sonority, and the tangible density that condense about us and penetrate us submerse us and buoy us up. Heidegger's antisubstantive ontology misses this sensuous density; for him the field is made of instrumental connections, and even the wind and the sunlight are grasped only in their serviceability and reliability[18]—and this layout of instrumental connections is suspended in the void.

The light, the sonority, and the tangible density that affect our moods engulf us, obturate our view, weigh down our hands with weariness or hold them in their vibrancy, such that we are embedded in the density that settles down upon us and survey very little.

Mood can sense not the instrumental layout as such, or the empty abysses, but the density of the light, the vibrancy of sonority, and the depths of the tangible. Mood may be subjection not to the whole space but to an isolated thing, when something does not so much focus our attention as weigh down upon us or engulf us and obturate our view, smothering the directions for an emotion. It is mood and not emotion we feel when our eyes do not circumscribe the possibilities in the forms of things but settle into their substance, when our eyes are lost in the depths of the ardent redness of the rose or the crystalline frailty of the wings of a dragonfly, when our ears are enchanted by the laughter of a woman or the five little notes Marcel Proust speaks of in *Swan's Way*, and when our hands are no longer gathering information or manipulating but drumming on the side of the bus or spreading the fluids of orgasm on the surfaces of a lover.

The holistic and temporal analysis of affectivity and understanding were intended by Heidegger to account for the direction of our actions. Understanding, which from the start envisions the environment comprehensively, would extend before the hand that reaches out a field of possibilities and a future. Affectivity, by which we find ourselves affected by the world in which we find ourselves, held by it, would retain behind us the past, and this implantation would give the starting point and the momentum of our movement. Heidegger went on to argue that the really possible is not extended by a representational mind that would diagram variants of the actual in front of it; the really possible is possibly impossible. Anxiety, the apprehensiveness before the impossible as such, before the abysses of nothingness and death, is the first understanding; it makes possible the apprehension of the presented as harboring possibilities. But Heidegger conceded that the premonition of the nothingness in which all that is possible is suspended cannot give direction to our movements. Beyond the brink of death there are no distances and no directions. More radically, there seems to be a confusion in the way Heidegger characterizes death temporally. He takes death to be the *Zu-kuft* which opens before us the whole field of the possible and the future. But anxiety is an anticipation rather than an expectation; death is not a future situated at the end of a line of time along which future events can be located, it is imminent, at each moment. Wherever one turns, death awaits.

In "Building Dwelling Thinking,"[19] Heidegger argues for the primacy of things that are locations, and of sites, that is, concrete layouts where the earth surfaces and the skies open, where mortals are assembled and sent forth to the beckonings of what is sacred, separated and wholesome. A location is not just a point; it is an assembling, a being that gathers earth and skies, mortals and harbingers of what is wholesome, and protects, preserves them in a site. It gives them a place, to take place. The establishing of a location is done by building in the twofold sense of assembling what does not come together of itself and caring for what grows of itself ("building up"). Heidegger shows that to build is to assemble something that itself assembles. A building is an assembler. In the essay "The Thing," he shows that a jug is not an assemblage of material and shape made by a human agent who first assembles in his mind the notion of the feast and the notion of the divinities, but that the jug assembles humans and the harbingers of the goodness, the sustenance of earth, and the energies of the skies.

Heidegger's late essays introduce *the divine*, formulated in the singular and in the neuter, but revealed in the world in the guise of the harbingers of the sacred, the "angels." The divine is not an ontological sphere transcendent to the world, but a constituent of the world. The world does not contain, in its space and time, the God or the goodness. But in the things in whose proximity we dwell—the jug and bench, the cross and crown, the heron and roe—there glow the traces of goodness. The existential movement by which the hand reaches out for things does not, then, open a great arc, encompassing the world, which returns to Dasein as the finality for which all things are means. The movement of the hand that builds for dwelling and dwells for building goes forth to the horizons and heights of the sacred, the separated, the goodness that draws as it withdraws. The mode in which the sacred affects us from the first is joy, Heidegger says, explicating Hölderlin. It is as mortals that we are anxiously drawn to things and through them to the goodness. It is not so much anxiety and courage, the dominant themes of authenticity in *Being and Time*, but anxiety and joy which are the ontological moods with which a world is given. There is no understanding of the sacred; the goodness is not a possibility grasped by powers; Heidegger refuses theodicy. It is poetry that chants the reverberations of the sacred in joy.

It would be then our proximity to things, and the joy that senses the traces of the sacred left on them, that would give direction to action and to our lives.

Locations are felt in moods, which weigh on us, affect us, engulf us, obturate our view. From these locations the positions of a life in space-time can be discerned. We think that it is the things considered not so much in their dynamic and instrumental forms but in their substance—their sensuous materiality that sustains and nourishes—that locations materialize. Do not the friends gathered in the tranquillity of the home encompassed by darkness leave aside the cares and tasks of the world, to lose themselves in the material substance of the jug and the liquor at rest within it?

The guerrillas have taken refuge in the peasant hut. The windows are shuttered; the kerosene lamp flickers feebly. They are silent. The farmer sets the jug of rum on the table and without saying anything takes a seat behind them. They do not speak to him about the ideology and the program for which they are fighting and being massacred, and in the name of which he who opened his door to them may tomorrow be tortured. They taste the almost forgotten savor of the rum. They do not thank him for his solidarity; nothing is said, they sit in the evidence of the naturalness of men partaking of the sap of the sugar canes aged in human toil. Here, this night, is the revolution, the utopia which so long seemed remote, lying beyond the socioeconomic analyses of ideology and beyond so many battles and fields of dead men. All that they have thought about, labored over, fought for, was that men, even in the most remote and most destitute corners of the land, partake together of the fruits of the earth. Here, this night, the revolution, the utopia, is there.

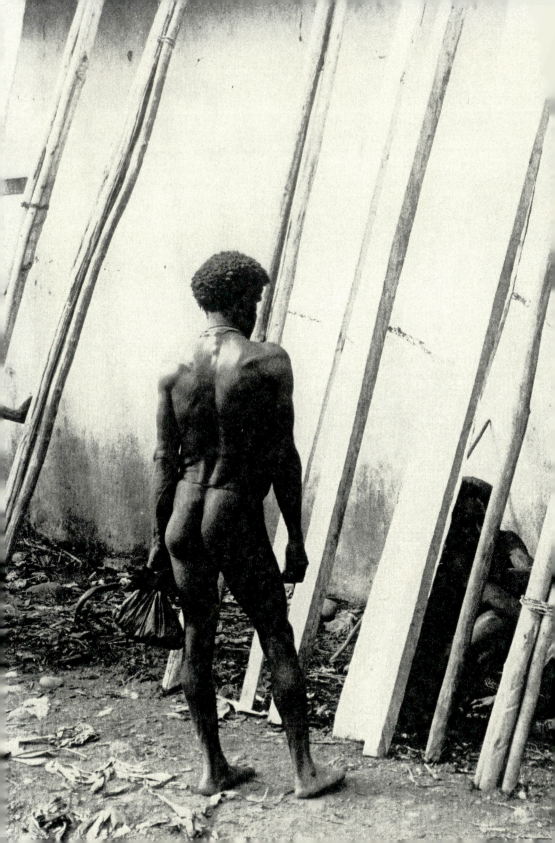

3

◆

Imperatives

All consciousness is consciousness of something; this Husserlian formula designates intentionality as the essence of consciousness. Is this "apodictic insight," like the laws of natural science, undecidably a law or a definition? The "something" in question toward which an awareness is intentionally turned is an object determined by scientific thought as empirically real; it is also a perceived pattern, a figment of the imagination, a proposition formulated in language, a number, the ego. But in perception, according to Maurice Merleau-Ponty's phenomenology, the something is a *thing*, an integrated, intersensorially consistent, graspable and manipulatable, real thing. The perception "devoted to things" shows that we exist in the world. A figure against a background—that is not a contingent trait of perception; it is the definition of perception, Merleau-Ponty writes at the beginning of *Phenomenology of Perception*.[1] Is this a psychological law, contingent then and admitting exceptions? Or is it a definition of what psychology will take to be perception?

Or is objective science, which represents objects, intrinsically dependent on the perception which presents things, such that it has to represent perception as presenting things? Then, why does science have to be objective, have to represent objects?

Merleau-Ponty finds, in the segmentation of the contemporary domain of sciences, a crisis in the very concept of objectivity. Conceptual models which reflect perceptual structures enter into the organization of the diverse segments of empirical research. Does this development show that the notion of *thing* rather than the notion of *object* is the imperative model for the scientific representation of the universe?

THE IMPERATIVES IN THINGS

The self that forms in our body, that sensitive-sensible *element* that moves itself, moves toward *things*. If a momentary pattern in the road is not confirmed

31

by more visibility, I doubt that I was really seeing; if a brief cry heard in the night is not followed by another sound or something visible, I doubt that there was anything and that I had heard. If, observing her more, I doubt that this woman has anything really engaging or seductive about her, I doubt the reality of my love. If, among the colors and sizes and shapes of things, my perception discerns the real properties from the colors, sizes, and shapes distorted by the medium, the distance, or the perspective; if I see the sheets of paper scattered on the floor under the desk as white even though they reflect light-waves objectively measurable as gray; if I see the snow in the troughs as white seen through blue shadow—it is because my perception is finalized toward seeing coherent and consistent things, maintaining their properties as they endure. I see a reflection not as a patch of gleaming color on the rim of the iris, but as an immaterial radiance playing over the sphere of the eye, which is brown and white. I feel as equally heavy two weights the one laid on my stomach, the other hung from my finger, though the weight of the one is distributed over a broad expanse of my body while that of the other is applied wholly upon a small area, and they are felt with two quite different systems of resistant tendons and muscles. I feel the grain and composition of the wood beneath the carved form of the statue which is felt as put on the subsistent ligneous substance. My perception is this power to attain from the first the intersensorial coherence and consistency of a thing, a transcendent ess-ence or way of being there, which no intersensorial exploration will ever make definitively given.

The distorted, phantom, or illusory appearances are distinguished in perception from the real properties because perception *has to* perceive things, coherent and consistent beings. The things *have to* not exhibit all their sides and qualities, have to compress them behind the faces they turn to us, have to tilt back their sides in depth, and not occupy all the field with their relative bigness, because they *have to* coexist in a field with one another, and that field *has to* coexist with the fields of the other possible things. The double monocular images dissipate as my eyes advance to the sight of a real thing; the visual form of a furry animal disappears and is not reworked and integrated into the form of the porous rock which materializes as I get closer. Some sensory patterns disconnect from the map of reality and float like phantoms before it, because they do not fit into the coherence and consistency of the world.

Seeing is believing; the visible form of a furry animal gave itself out as a pattern in the world and in the real, but not as the real or true being itself; it was provisional, attendant upon confirmation through more seeing. The apparition of the real is not composed out of such appearances, for when I step closer it dissipates to give place to the more dense apparition of the porous rock.[3] Yet real or true being is not something apart from these always presumptive appearances, since what motivates the dissociation of the furry animal from the real world is not an apprehension of the logic and necessities of the field, but the subsequent apparition in its place of the rock whose visibility persists. The "belief" in the reality of the first appearance is "revoked" only by being transferred to the next. More exactly, there are not successive acts of judgment; one takes as real the consistent appearance that forms on the sensible levels of the world.

The world in which we perceive extends in a space-time that is not a priori apprehendable in the formulas for Euclidean or nonEuclidean geometrical dimensions and the objective time of successive moments. It extends on *levels*— the level of the light which our gaze adjusts to and sees with as it looks at the illuminated contours that surface and intensify, the level of the sonority our hearing attunes to as it harkens to sounds and noises that rise out of it, the level of the tangible our posture finds as our limbs move across the contours and textures of tangible substances, the level of verticality and of depth and of rest that emerges as our position becomes functional in a layout of tasks.[4] The level is found sensorially, by a movement that does not grasp at it as an objective but adjusts to it, is sustained by it, moves with it and according to it.

The duration of the perceived world also has to be conceived as a level. The time of the world is not a dimension *t+1* projected by a conceptual operation, in which we locate the present moment in which all that is perceivable is presented. The future and the past extend like horizons, not horizons we view but levels on which we find ourselves embarked and that sustain the configuration of the present. Our perceiving organism presents itself in the course of the world, and the present moment it determines is not a closed form that reproduces itself along a linear dimension but a relief on a level of futurity and passage. The future extends not as a unit about to displace the present moment but as a directive toward which and with which we turn. The present as it passes does not subsist in the form of a closed moment that has, as Husserl put it, undergone simply the modification of distance; it loses its particularity, veers into generality, is no longer before us as the object of perception or the object of recall but becomes the angle and the momentum with which we now envision what is there.

The world is not a framework, an order, or an arrangement, but a nexus of levels. The levels are not dimensions we can survey from above; we find them not by moving toward them but by moving with them. A level is determinate not as an extension we can survey or a periodicity we can diagram, but as a style we catch on to by moving with it and catching on to how each scene and each moment varies the last and launches a variation in its turn—as we catch on to the style of a writer or of a conversation not by understanding the axioms from which each proposition is being derived, but by catching on to the rhythm, the tempo, the scope of the shifts, and the range of the variations and repartees. The world holds together the fields in which we perceive in a consistency and coherence which is not formulable as a set of universal laws, but apprehended as a style caught on the move and engendering variants by which we recognize the visible, the tangible, the sonorous realms beneath the monocular images, the will-o'-the-wisps, and the mirages.

The reality of the sensible levels, of the world—which is not the evidence of constitutional laws and necessities—gives to any thing in the world the evidence of its being real. The apparition of the sensible world is not that of a true representation, since all of the beings it presents and contains are given as real contingent upon subsequent perceptual confirmation, and since the coherence and compossibility of the fields of our various senses and of the transtemporal and intercorporeal field is never given and formulable, but is known only in the continuous transitions by which each field opens upon the next.[5] But the reality of the sensible field is not effectively doubtable, since every doubt we can have and every disillusioning we can experience concerns only particular configurations within it, and we doubt the reality of any appearance only by believing more in another perceptible configuration.[6] Any more intelligible or more coherent representation we could have of the universe, including that of the universe of fully determinate objectivity which we posit as the ideal term of all our scientific investigations, could not be more certain or more real than the field we perceive, for every such representation is a re-presentation, in the linguistic formulations and calculus of our reason, of the field of our perception, and has to verify its calculations of what is real by controlled observations of the perceivable.

THE WORLD AS AN IMPERATIVE

What then is this finality that makes our perception *have to* perceive things and *have to* perceive a field of compossible things, a world? It is not a determinism; we can see without inevitably seeing things and without necessarily seeing a world. We can see monocular images and not binocular visions of things; our eyes can get caught up in phantasms and pre-things, in the caricatural doubles and mirages the sensible levels and planes also engender. Our look can record only the contours and finish our desires and our obsessions, our loves and our hatreds have put on the nodes in the fabric of sensible reality; our eyes and our hands can touch only the shapings culture and industry have left on the levels of the natural world. We can take refuge from the planes of sensible reality in a dream-space; we can drag fragments of things into a delirious space without levels and consistent dimensions; we can, as in advanced states of melancholia, settle in the realm of death.[7]

The things subsist not as givens, but as tasks to which perception finds itself devoted. A thing arises as a relief on the levels of the world which extend about it and harbor other things, to which this thing turns its lateral sides; these outlying things invite us as standpoints from which those sides can be seen. To reach the other sides of a thing before us, we have to displace ourselves to those other standpoints in the landscape the other things mark out for us. The levels extend the world as a system where the things witness one another and each contributes to the consistency and coherence of all. The thing ordering the direction of our perception leads us to the consistency and coherence of the levels; the levels which we can reach only by subjecting ourselves to them conduct us to things. The things are not given in perception but order it as tasks; the world, nexus of levels, exists not as a perceptual given but as an imperative.

The directives with which the world extends are not given in perceptual presentation, nor in conceptual representation. The world is not given in the consistency and coherence of a saturated set of universal and necessary laws. We cannot derive the position and structure of the things emerging in the course of the world out of a blueprint our theory can represent. As we turn toward a thing we do see sketched out on the side it turns to us prefigurations of its other sides, and we see about it the other things whose consistency witnesses those other sides; but to reach those other sides we have to displace ourselves to see it from the standpoints the surrounding things fix for us, and in the time the displacement takes the side we have now left behind may discolor, bulge or shrivel, or disintegrate. Our very exploratory movements about it leave their marks on it. It would take an indefinite expanse of time to make each of its sides face us—and each thing the course of the world presents disintegrates in the course of time. A thing is before us as a task and a reality embedded in the subsistence of the world inasmuch as it is closed in itself and harbors secrets and surprises. The world-order which sustains it, the levels which maintain it, are presented not as a framework surveyed but as directives pursued. The very representation we formulate, the set of formulations with which we represent its coherence and consistency as universal and necessary laws, is the way our theoretical reason seeks to follow its imperatives.

THE A PRIORI EXTERIORITY OF THE IMPERATIVE

The imperative from which all hypothetical imperatives derive their imperative force is as a fact. It is the first fact. Kant argued that it is the imperative laid on thought to think consistently and coherently that makes empirical facts recognizable as facts. The ultimately imperative is ungroundable and unrepresentable. The imperative itself is not a principle the mind would formulate or a program the mind would set before itself in a representation. Every principle with which reason represents what is imperative is constituted by a mind that is bound already to think according to principles. The imperative is not, as in Heidegger's interpretation of Kant,[8] the program the mind would formulate of a project that our existence is. The force of the imperative is prior to the representation with which one makes its formulation present before oneself. The imperative weighs on the mind as an exteriority prior to the exteriority of the world of extended objects it presents.

Kant argues that thought is itself the original locus of the imperative. He explains that the consistency and coherence of the phenomenal field derives from the ordering activity of the understanding which combines with sensation to produce perception of objects, and from the ordering activity of reason which relates coexisting and successive objects. Thought which understands correctly and reasons rightly is thought which represents coherence and consistency—which represents objects according to their universal and necessary structure and represents the coexistence and succession of objects according to their universal and necessary order. Thought can think something, can actualize itself as thought, only by thinking according to the universal and the necessary. This imperative is not a psychological necessity, which could be explained by representing the innate structure and determined relationship between the psychic apparatus and its objective environment. Such an explanation would itself be a work of thought, and would have already presupposed that thought subjected to the imperative, in order to be consistent and coherent. As soon as thought thinks, it finds itself subjected to an imperative to represent the universal and the necessary. Thought is obedience. But it must command the perception and the motility that collect content for its ordering activity. Thought is commanded to be in command.

For Merleau-Ponty, thought finds itself commanded to think the consistent and the coherent because it is destined to think of real things and the real world.[9] Thought is not constitutive of perception; it is a representation of the layout of things presented in perception. It is not only the content of things but their forms that command thought. The imperative laid on the receptivity of the spontaneity of understanding is itself grounded on the imperative laid on a sensibility that can actualize itself as perception only by being receptive to the levels and ordering axes of the world and perceiving things compossible within the world. Perception seeks in the sensorial patterns things which direct its intentionality, and pursues the levels in which they are arrayed and which command it as an ordinance. The subjection of the mind to an imperative is first the subjection of perception to the imperatives in things and the imperative ordinance of the world. It is the subjection of the subject to the exterior not as a material pressure which affects its sensory surfaces as sensations and affects its movements as reactions, but as an ordinance which directs the intentional focus of its sensory powers and its exploratory positions and movements. The imperative is first in the world, to which the sensitive-sensible flesh finds itself ordered, prior to any formation of dream-images, appearances that are not appearances of things, desiderata, implement-structures, or organizing principles for its representations. The exteriority of the force of the imperative, not presented in the mind that represents the formulation of law it commands, is the exteriority of the world. It is the world not as a multiplicity of identifiable things a posteriori affecting the mind, but as an ordinance a priori laid on the mind. Or, more exactly, laid on our existence, which exists as destined for the world.

THE IMPERATIVE IS PRACTICAL

For Kant, the imperative is elucidated as an imperative for rational autonomy. The imperative, first seated in the understanding, commands thought to actualize itself, commands it to be in command, to command the sensory-motor organs that collect content for thought, and to disengage the activating will in our composite sensible nature from the lures of objects given as sensuous. As our practical powers manipulate things, they must arrange them not as so many sensuous lures but as intelligible structures. The imperative, as an imperative laid on a composite agency, becomes an imperative to act on the phenomenal field so as to order external nature in conformity with the rational representation of the universe, which thought constitutes in obedience to its own a priori imperative. Reason, then, by virtue of its own imperative, has to become practical.

For Merleau-Ponty, the world-imperative is received not on our understanding in conflict with our sensuality, but on our postural schema which integrates our sensibility and mobilizes our efficacity. The world-imperative commands our sensibility first to realize itself, as a praktognosis oriented to things. It commands our sensitive-sensible body to inhabit a world of things with the most centered, integral, and efficacious hold, from which every subsequent kind of comprehension will be derived. It orders our competence.

For perception is praktognosis.[10] Perceived things are objectives. To perceive one has to look, one has to mobilize oneself and manipulate one's surroundings. To see a visible thing in real space is to feel how to get to it and how to handle it. The moon, as it rises over the planes and paths of the landscape in which I circulate, loses its determinate color and size, the mountain which I never address with a body intention of climbing floats as a phantom over reality; they become ultra-things, as Wallon classifies them, like the phantom monocular images a motor intentionality mobilizing both eyes as one organ has not solidified into one integral vision of one thing. Sensation itself is behavior: to sense the green and the blue is to adopt a certain posture and to contract a certain muscular tonus;[11] to hear a sound is to turn to it and to follow it. To synthesize the information collected on the diverse sense organs is to synergically center one's surfaces and members and organs upon it. It is with a movement of one's hand that one perceives the texture and the grain of a surface; it is with a posture of one's mobile body that one perceives the position of a thing in the landscape, its up-down axis, its *sens*—its meaning and its orientation.[12] Each perceived thing is a task and a means toward locating the next thing. Each profile of a thing is an objective for a body that has to center itself and a means for grasping the coherence and cohesion of something.

The engagement in the world, which is not a determination but an imperative, admits also a movement of disengagement from the sensible fields and levels of the world. "The relation between the things and my body is decidedly singular; it is what makes me sometimes remain in appearances, and it is also what sometimes brings me to the things themselves; it is what produces the buzzing of appearances, it is also what silences them and casts me fully into the world. Everything comes to pass as though my power to reach the world and my power to entrench myself in phantasms only came one with the other; even more, as though the access to the world were but the other face of a withdrawal and this retreat to the margin of the world a servitude and another expression of my natural power to enter into it."[13] The body that advances down and retreats from the levels at which things are found is the competent body, which can have objectives because the futures and possibilities of things are open-ended and because the imperative that makes each thing an objective is relativized by the next thing, and because the levels do not hold him unless he takes hold of them. The disengagement from the world is constitutive of its competence.

THE OBJECTIVE IMPERATIVE

The theoretical representation of the universe elaborated by science is a representation of the perceived environment, which is not an amorphous medley of sensory givens but a field of things which emerge as tasks, ordinances commanding our postural focus, along levels which regulate our advance. The perceptual field is practicable, open to the initiatives of our sensory-motor powers, and open too to the manipulations, isolations, and experimentations by which the theorist selects and observes his data; it is open to the instruments the theorist uses to refine his substances and engineer his verifications. Theoretical practices are but one group among the larger number of initiatives our practical powers take in the perceptual field, to advance into it, to uncover things, to bring their possibilities and relationships to light. Empiricism in science means that every theoretical entity one constructs remains but hypothetical, an instrument of calculation, until it enables one to make predictions which are verified by observation, that is, by perceivable events in a practicable field. Atoms, electromagnetic fields, gravity—these are theoretical constructs which are not more real than the rocks, trees, birds, and fishes; they are theoretical instruments to represent the observed relationships between rocks, trees, birds, and fishes. Science does not find that the solidity and color of the rock is merely apparent; the subatomic particles moving at enormous velocity have as their sole justification the reactions one observes on the perceived rock. If one were to doubt that the rocks, trees, birds, and fishes were real, one would revoke into doubt at the same time the theoretical entities constructed by the natural scientists.

Science remains empirical when its theoretical elaborations, its microphysics, and its cosmology constructed perhaps for decades without experimental verification, one day programs the technological production of the prostheses that enormously expand the sphere of what is perceivable with the sense organs with which the human species has been genetically and culturally endowed. It remains empirical when the constructions with purely theoretical entities and with mathematics now cut absolutely free of their original moorings in geography and architecture design the technology that will equip the scientific observer to see like eagles and wasps, perceive with the sonar echolocation of bats and the sixth sense of fish, navigate with the magnetic or cosmic sense of migratory birds and insects, and discern infinitesimal vibrations with the sensitivity of single cells or single electrons in those bats and fish.

Scientific observation does not only supersede natural perception to reach with the prosthetic organs technology has devised a more minute, more precise, and more stable percept; in recording its observations, it converts the percept into an *object*.[14] The percept given in scientific observation is relocated in geometrical space and metric time, indifferent to its contents, in which the object figures as the subsistent substrate of all its forms and attributes which observation finds in the varying perspectives of the perceived field and at different moments of a wave of duration. The object is the simultaneous realization in a segment of cosmic time of all the aspects and facets that the perspectival and successive exploration of a thing will make determinate. While real things in the perceived world are reliefs whose determinations form and eclipse across a wave of duration, the objects that furnish the scientific representation of the universe are represented as fully determined at each instant of their existence.

The scientist sets out to objectify his own body, with which he observes the perceived world. He will set out to do, over the time it takes, a complete itemization of all the contents and events of his body, and realize them simultaneously in an objective representation of his organism. He will set out to determine precisely the correlations between events in this object and the other determinate events of the objective environment.

About our bodies, now represented as objects in the midst of other objects in the objective representation of the universe, there is produced a field of perceived appearances, in which the surrounding things appear not as objects but as open-ended things forming on levels. The empirical psychologist will make observations of this perceptual field and record an objective version of it. He will determine its parameters, he will record the patterns that take form within it, analyze its simplest component elements, which he takes to be elementary sense-data, or sensations. He will then set out to correlate each point of color in the visual field with a physiological stimulus on the retina and nerve paths of the eye. He will show how physical events in the outside environment send physico-chemical and electromagnetic stimuli upon the organism; he will record the physiological impulses in the afferent and efferent nervous circuitry of the objective body. He will then show how, projected in the brain, these physiological impulses result in psychic events, spots of color composing patterns in the visual field. The perceived patterns will be represented as effects of psychophysiological events in the objective body. The perceptual field will then figure as a segment of the objective representation of the universe. The empirical psychophysiologist will have determined how the objects of the external universe—the objects in his representation of the universe—produce that image of themselves which is the representation of the environment produced in perception.

There will remain for the cognitive psychologist to determine how the sensations associate among themselves according to psychological laws and produce general configurations, and how abstract concepts result from the association of sensations in the mind. He will one day determine how his mind produces out of its representation of the outside objects which is the perceptual field that second representation which is his objective representation of the universe. This psychology which constructs the world justifies itself with every advance in neurophysiology which maps on the neural substance of the organism localizations of the sensations with which the world is represented. It would explain the world-order ultimately by the physiological imperatives of our own organism.

At the limit, the scientific theorist will produce one total objective representation of the universe, comprising an objective representation of all outside things given through perception, an objective representation of the scientist's own body that perceives those things, an objective representation of the scientist's own mind in which a perceptual field is produced representing in sensorial patterns a segment of the universe about that scientist, and a representation of the processes by which that scientist's mind produces his very science and his objective representation of all things.

But Merleau-Ponty argues that the theoretical objective, to represent the things we observe as objects and the field opened by our perception as an objective universe, is itself motivated by the structure of things which command our perception. To perceive is for my gaze to go out of my location to where the thing is, to inhabit it as it shows itself. On the contours of the side it turns to me I see adumbrated the other sides of that thing, sides it turns to things located alongside of it and behind it. My gaze is refracted to those places occupied by those other things, and already goes there to envision the thing from their positions. As each thing draws my gaze into its reality, it implants itself in a setting extended by the levels that support it and where the other things on those levels designate other perceivable sites from which it is perceivable. I do not only see the thing with the levels, with the light, with the verticality and repose of the field, but I see it with the other things which mark out viewing points on those levels. When I look at the giant sequoia before me, my vision attributes to it the other sides as they would be seen by the other trees about it, by the hills beyond and the river below and the clouds above; each of these other things, visible and real and a possible location for my look, guarantees for this tree the reality of all the sides now turned away from my gaze. This is the experience that makes me see each side of the thing as determinate: all its sides are kept determinate by the determinate forms of the other things of the world.

When I enter the luminous space of a room and look at this desk before me, presenting itself, establishing a moment of presence, it looks like it was there a moment ago and will be there in another moment. When the desk presents itself it also presents how it will go on being, how it was already. Something instantaneous, utterly unanticipatable and that vanishes at once, is a mirage, a phantom; it could not present itself as real. Each moment in which something is presented does not give itself out as the instantaneous correlate of my arising there and presenting myself. Each moment of duration invokes, as its witnesses to anticipate and to confirm its presence, past and future moments. When I look at what is presented, I look out into the moments behind and ahead of it. The things appear embedded in the continuation of time; each present moment appears as fixed and identifiable in the interconnected moments of the course of the world.

Each thing that presents itself thus invites us to view it as something crystallized in a world of other things crystallized about it, in a fixed and identifiable moment on the axis of the time of the world. Each thing invites us to situate it not within the hold of our body centered on it, but within the system of the world and within the axis of its interlocked moments. Our own position, our own approach to it appear incidental to its being there.

This incipient perceived closure that directs perception to things is what motivates the scientific project of representing each thing as totally determinate now, within a universal system of outlying things also fully determinate now. It is what motivates the project of objectification, which represents the world presented in perception without levels extending indefinitely and without things exhibiting open-ended consistency in a time that can contain surprises. Objectification eliminates from the representation of reality the structure of one determinate figure against a less determinate or indeterminate background, and represents the light, darkness, heat, sonority, rumble, and silence in which things are found as themselves completely determinate multiplicities of completely determinate objects.

What the objectifying project of empirical science does is carry out the determination of each thing by the surrounding things, each moment by the preceding and following moments, all the way to the limit. In doing so it is commanded by the imperative that rules our perceptual life, which orients our perception toward the positing of things and of the coexistence of things.

THE APORIA

Merleau-Ponty's phenomenology makes perception a praktognosis, makes our existence a stand whose posture is directed upon objectives, makes our body occupied and laborious. He argues that the representation science elaborates of the objective universe is itself motivated by the imperative world-levels which present things as objectives for competent bodies. Objective science is not only a practical project in that the theorist refines his substances and engineers his verifications with manipulations, isolations, and experimentations. Its objects themselves are objectives that represent the tasks things are for perception.

Yet the objectified representation of the universe is no longer a practicable world. The objective representation of the universe elaborated by science represents beings as in themselves totally determinate; it is a representation that renders as present their past and their future appearances. The sensible pivots are stabilized into points, the levels converted into lines, the horizons into planes, the depths into volumes, the space between things into potentially observable things, the murmur of silence into a multiplicity of tones. The body is converted into an exhaustively observable object determined from all points of view, where excitations in principle locatable at each moment as they travel the nervous circuitry result in temporally locatable psychic facts. Objective psychology represents the field of experience which that body maintains about itself as completely determinate, decomposable into psychic facts, sensations, which are in a constant relationship with the objective properties of external stimuli. Eventually the psychophysiologist would have to explain in terms of determinate correlations his own thought processes by which he produces the scientific representation of psychic facts, just as the physicist produces his representation of the external stimuli. The objective scientist represents his body as an object agitated by outside forces triggering the ends of its nervous circuitry, and represents his own perceptual field and his objectified representation of the universe itself as ultimately produced by those outside objects. The theorist who has converted the world of levels with which he perceives into a representation of fully determinate objects whose perceptual possibilities are actualized, whose future apparitions are present, and who has converted the ipseity that forms in the reciprocal inscription of postural schema and body image into a representation of a psychophysical object, locates himself everywhere and nowhere; he converts himself into a high-altitude absolute subject contemplating a body-object he no longer moves with. The original imperative that ordered a field of experience about him was laid on his body as a system of practical powers; when this imperative is carried out to the limit by the project of objectifying the universe, the scientist's own body, and the scientist's own mind, end in a total disengagement from every practicable field, including the field of that praxis which is empirical observation.

This disengagement from the world is itself commanded by the world-imperative. "Human life 'understands' not only a certain definite environment, but an infinite number of possible environments, and it understands itself because it is thrown into a natural world. Human behavior opens upon a world (*Welt*) and upon an object (*Gegenstand*) beyond the tools which it makes for itself, and one may even treat one's own body as an object. Human life is defined in terms of this power which it has of denying itself in objective thought, a power which stems from its primordial attachment to the world itself."[15]

THE SEGMENTATION OF THE THEORETICAL UNIVERSE

The pursuit of the objective imperative issues in a split from the practicable field in which theoretical research must nonetheless effect its observations and its verifications. But Merleau-Ponty also sees in the science of our day the objective universe separating into discontinuous segments.

Psychology discovers, by its own methods, the unverifiability of the hypothesis of a constant relationship between physiological impulses and the gestalts that form in the subject's field of perception. The region-specific concepts which it formulates to record those gestalts are unconvertible into the concepts that record physiological processes. Physiology discovers, by its own methods, that the behavior of a living organism is correlative not with the objective properties of the external objects impinging upon it but with their phenomenal properties. It discovers it must, to understand behavior, correlate it not with the objective representation of the universe elaborated in physics, but with the sensory appearance of its environment which the organism itself elaborates with the sense organs specific to it. The physiological environment presented to an organism disconnects from the physical universe represented by the physicist. Eventually, physics too discovers, as ultimate physical facts, relational events which implicate the observer in the observed. The physical universe closes in about the physicist and disconnects from his own physiological environment and his field of perception.

The segmentation of the objective representation of the universe is fixed with the introduction of region-specific concepts and organizational models. Merleau-Ponty's phenomenology of perception was a theoretical project intended to fix a set of descriptive, and not objectifying, concepts and organizational models specific for the perceived field. Merleau-Ponty's thesis is that the new region-specific models we find in the physical, the physiological, the psychological, and the cognitive-science segments of contemporary science are likewise descriptive and not objectifying concepts and organizational models. And that they are in fact derived from the concepts and organizations specific to the field of perception. Not only in fact: obligatorily. For his thesis is that the scientific representation of the universe finds itself obliged, at a certain point in its elaboration, to return to the perceived world, not only to verify its calculations but to remodel its concepts.[16] And this imperative is intrinsically practical.

Merleau-Ponty's phenomenology of perception demonstrates that it was able to elaborate descriptive concepts with which we can identify the structures specific to perceptual things, those open-ended sensuous essences, which could not exist apart from the perceiving bodies for which their colors, their textures, their weights are real, and which could not exist as real things except by being always beyond what we grasp of them or determine of them. The phenomenology of perception was able to describe the real world in terms of levels, and to differentiate this concept from the concepts of dimension, framework, and order. It was able to describe the perceiver not as a psychophysiological object programmed by a priori concepts, but as a postural schema mobilized by perceived things and engendering a body-image of itself as a thing among things.

In the scientific representation of the universe today, we find concepts akin to these descriptive concepts.[17] This development is most advanced in physics. When physics insists that what it can record is what it can operate on with its instruments and its mathematics, it is defining physical entities not as absolute objects but as correlates of our operations. Einstein's theory of general relativity and the Heisenberg uncertainty principle force the physicist to take as his ultimate entities not pure objects but relationships between observer and observed. The physicist no longer takes simultaneity or succession as absolutes, univocally determinable. Physics today admits horizonal phenomena, properties without substances, collective entities or pure multiplicities, entities without simple location.

In his first book *The Structure of Behavior*,[18] Merleau-Ponty traced a similar transformation in contemporary physiology. Empirical physiology was first based on anatomy. One analytically decomposed the body and set out to determine with precision all its component elements. The behavior of the body was broken down into elementary reflex arcs, and one sought to correlate these with elementary physico-chemical or electromagnetic stimuli, and to explain a movement, a gesture, or an operation as the sum of a multiplicity of these automatic reflex arcs. This attempt at an analytic explanation did not succeed. The sensory thresholds, which determine at any moment the intensity and force of a stimulus that would release a reflex arc, are variable, and they vary according to the posture, the centering, the metabolic state of the whole organism. When our bodies are centered on a task in front of us, the sensory thresholds on our back are higher; it takes more pressure, more intense cold or heat on our back before we feel it. The innervation of our hand at any phase of a movement cannot be put in a one-to-one correlation with external stimuli; it is, like a molecule of soap on the surface of an expanding bubble, determined by the configuration of the whole, by the scope and sweep and rhythm of the gesture. Each step we take is not only determined by the contours of the terrain and by the air pressure, but also by the gait, that is, the general rhythm we maintain when we launch our bodies into a continuous advance. We have to envision the position and movement of each of our parts not in function simply of the external pressures bombarding them but also in function of the postural axes they maintain and vary, in function of the gait they maintain, in function of the total diagram of a gesture, of an operation. In order to determine the physiological functioning of our body parts, our limbs, organs, glands, our body chemistry and electrical fields, we have to envision our bodies as systems that do not tend to a state of rest like inanimate things, but tend to maintain certain typical levels of tension, which are in correlation with the typical tasks our bodies maintain themselves in readiness for. We have to envision the functional organism not with the microscopic focus of the anatomist, but with a focus that takes in the whole posture of the organism and its correlates in its perceived environment. The concepts of posture, gesture, and coordinated movement with which physiological behavior is theoretically represented are concepts derived from the way physiological behavior appears in the perceptual field of the physiologist, and do not constitute an objective replacement for it.

The project of an objective psychology has likewise been transformed. The hypothesis of constancy, of a constant relationship between psychic sensations and physiological impulses and physical stimuli, could not be verified. It was found that the patterns that form in our field of perception could not be correlated with constellations of physical stimuli. Colors that form in our field of vision by contrast have no corresponding physical reality. The figure-ground organization of our field of perception does not correspond to anything physical on the retinas of our eyes. Distinctive regional concepts will be introduced to identify the typical patterns and structures within the field of perception. These concepts will no longer be objectifying, but descriptive of the open-ended structures of things as they appear in perception and of the levels of the perceived field which are not the dimensions in which objects are located.

The psychologist, in the name of the rigor of his own discipline, ends up describing the psychic field as a complex of nonobjects, appearances of open-ended things. The physiologist ends up not explaining the positions and movements of organisms by events in his objective representation of the universe, but correlating the postures, gestures, and operations of an organism as they appear in the field of perception of the physiologist and as they appear to that organism itself with the open-ended things that figure in the perceptual field of that organism. The specific structures of perceptual patterns and levels show through in the objects and dimensions of physics. Objectifying science was a praxis that would have ended up constituting a representation of the universe that made praxis inconceivable, but on the way finds that its representation of the objective universe re-presents the practicable format of the world of perception. The cognitive psychology that set out to explain the concepts of science itself as events in the objective universe ends up inscribing them in the field of postures and gestures. The scientist, motivated by the imperatives in things and in the practicable world to devote himself to elaborating an objectifying representation of the universe, finds himself returning to a world of sensible levels in order to understand how he is commanded to pursue objectification, what operations his thought effects on the things given in his phenomenal field, and how he occupies a viewpoint, stands, moves, and sees.

INTERPRETING THE PRIMACY OF PERCEPTION

Merleau-Ponty then argues that there is nonetheless a universal field which contains all the segmented domains of empirical research. This field is not the universal form of objectivity; it is the perceived world. The region theoretically delimited as the physico-chemical sphere, that delimited as the physiological sphere, that delimited as the psychological sphere, and that delimited as the cognitive sphere are in fact all theoretically elaborated representations of sectors of the perceived sphere. The argument is not only that they draw their data from empirical observation, that is, from perceptions; it is also that the general form of all their new concepts reflects perceptual diagrams of apprehension. It is concepts, the identifying and organizing concepts that are region-specific, that segment an empirical domain from the continuity of nature. But if all these concepts are perception-derived, they should make possible a new continuity between the empirical regions they organize and segment.

Merleau-Ponty has linked the imperatives in things with the imperative the world is. The things arise as reliefs on the levels of the world which extend about them and harbor other things to which they turn their lateral sides and which invite us as standpoints from which those sides can be seen. The levels extend the world as a network of directives conducting us to things and to settings made of things. The thing ordering the direction of our perception leads us to the consistency and coherence of the levels; the levels which we can reach only by subjecting ourselves to them conduct us to things. The levels pursued in whatever direction also lead us back to the things from which we started. When the music we are engrossed in comes to an end, we pick up the thread of the world again as when we awaken to the visible again which continued uninterrupted during the interval of our sleep. As for Kant the imperative is inseparable from the form of universality and necessity, for Merleau-Ponty the imperative is inseparable from the consistency and coherence of one world. Our new scientific competencies, our prostheses technologically devised, which open up new theaters in the space of the world, are continuous with the sensory-motor competency that dedicates our perception to things, and to which the competent scientific observer returns.

The argument seems to us to have weak points. To argue that all theoretical regions are theoretically elaborated representations of sectors of the perceived sphere which for its part is one and encompassing is to argue that everything empirically observed is located on the levels of the perceived landscape. It is to argue that it is only its re-presentation that relocates it on the axes of another space. Yet microscopic and macroscopic science has not only made more clear and distinct the things of the perceivable field, not only articulated the horizons of that field, but changed its shape and its time. If it is true that scientific observation differs from natural perception in that it narrows its focus, sets up its own controls, and determines what will count as verification, is it not also true that scientific observation segments, isolates, disconnects the field in which its perception is made from the levels of the natural world?

One transforms not only the hue, but the substance and location of a color by changing the focus of one's look, reorganizing the scope of the field. Conversely, in transforming the clarity and distinctness of a perceived pattern does one not disconnect its space from the space of the world? When one views a segment of the wall through a tube, it loses its hue, its density, and its surface and becomes a thin medium extending before the eye. The moon, whose size could be gauged when seen through a tube, loses any measurable size when seen in the open sky. When one ceases to perceive the tones rumbling in the horns and on the skins of the drums and follows them as they relate to one another, the space of the music disconnects from the visual space bounded by the walls of the concert hall. When, after the piece is played the lights go on in the hall and one returns to the world of the visible and of things, one shakes one's head as though awakening from a dream.

The objective representation of the universe programs the technology to contrive the prostheses that will enable the scientific observer, equipped by nature and by prior culture with only the sense organs specific to the human organism, to observe the data that would justify the theoretical hypotheses, and also to open new regions for exploration. The space of the micro- or macrophysicist, accessible through his prostheses, is not observable with the practices of the biologist; the space the biologist maps out is not observable with the practices of the psychologist; the space where the psychologist finds his data is not observable with the methods of the cognitive scientist. These new regions of data annexed to the world given to prescientific perception show structures that are, if not those of absolute determination in geometrical space and linear time in which objects are represented, also not those of the levels and durations in which the things of prescientific perception are found. Is not the segmentation of the theoretical representation of the universe also a segmentation of the regions of observation and a segmentation of the observing organism?

Would we not have to argue that the segmentation of the scientific representation of the world reflects a segmentation already at work in the world of perception, and a discontinuity in our competencies? If the new descriptive concepts and organizational concepts Merleau-Ponty has pointed to in the diverse regions of contemporary science are indeed so many abstract diagrams of perceptual syntheses and perceptual synergies, they are not simply variants of the things of prescientific perception and of the synergic postures with which those things are approached. To observe scientifically one has to develop new competencies, and one equips oneself with prostheses devised by technology. One obeys new imperatives.

The eyes that have to dissipate the monocular image and reach the thing have to "act as the two channels of a single Cylopian vision;" the sensory-motor apparatus that has to dissipate the flux of reflections and shadows, perspectival deformations, and mirages to come to grips with things has to "do but one thing at a time," has to stand and to move as a synergic and focused whole. The prostheses-equipped competencies of scientific observers become those of the eyes of eagles and wasps, of the sonar echolocation of bats and the sixth sense of fish, of the magnetic or cosmic sense of migratory birds and insects, of the sensitivity of single cells or single electrons in those bats and fish. The imperatives that scientists find in the micro- and macrocosmic theaters they enter are no longer the imperatives the natural perception of our species found in things. These imperatives are recognized and obeyed with other competencies that those which enable our bodies to perceive things.

THE IMPERATIVE INCOMPETENCE

Is competence alone imperative? What of the disengagement from things, and from the levels and planes which engender things, toward those refuges from the space of the world where the phantom doubles of monocular vision, perceptual illusions, mere appearances refract off the surfaces of things? What of the dream-scene, the private theaters of delirious apparitions, that realm of death in which the melancholic takes up his abode? What of the possibility of releasing one's hold on the levels, drifting into a sensible apeiron without levels, into that nocturnal, oneiric, erotic, mythogenic second space that shows through the interstices of the daylight world of praktognostic competence?

We would argue that the world in Merleau-Ponty's sense—the light that forms a level along which color-contrasts phosphoresce, the key about which the melody rises and falls, the murmur of nature from which a cry rises, the rumble of the city beneath which a moan of despair descends—these levels themselves form in a medium without dimensions or directions—the luminosity more vast than any panorama that the light outlines in it, the vibrancy that prolongs itself outside the city and beyond the murmur of nature, the darkness more abysmal than the night from which the day dawns and into which it confides itself. Is not the world, in Merleau-Ponty's sense, itself set in depths, in uncharted abysses, where there are vortices in which the body that lets loose its hold on the levels of the world, the dreaming, visionary, hallucinating, or lascivious body, gets drawn, and drags with it not things, but those appearances without anything appearing, those phantoms, caricatures, and doubles that even in the high noon of the world float and scintillate over the contours of things and the planes of the world?

But we also think that if the sensibility is drawn into these vortices beyond the nexus of levels where the world offers things, it is drawn imperatively. Does not the visionary eye that is not led to the lambent things the light of the world illuminates obey another imperative in the light—the imperative to shine? Does not the vertigo that gives itself over to the abyss that descends and descends without end obey not the imperative of the depth to maintain surfaces, but another imperative that depth promotes and is: to deepen? Does not the hearing that hears not the particular songs, cries, and noises of the world, but the vibrancy beyond the corridors of the world, obey the imperative of hearing that it become vibrant?

And what of the imperative not to hold onto things and maintain the world, but to release every hold and to lose the world, an imperative which everyone who has to die knows? There is in Merleau-Ponty's *Phenomenology of Perception* no word of this, only the imperative figure of an agent that holds onto things that are objectives and that maintains himself or herself in the world. One dies of the world, and one dies into the world. The competence of the body casts it fully into the world and brings it to the things themselves; has not this competence also been a sending forth of its sensibility and its motor force into them, a taking leave of itself? In committing itself to them, does it not also disengage from them, and from its own powers, from its competence?

Heidegger had recognized the having to die with all one's own forces to be our very nature, but he equates it, dialectically, and to us incomprehensibly, with the resolute and caring hold on things and on the world. The care for things, the perception devoted to the sensible patterns that pass, is not only a presumptive apprehension of their integrated, intersensorially consistent, graspable and manipulatable, real structures. It is also a movement that lets the patterns pass, the reliefs merge into levels, the configurations dissolve into light and resonance and terrestrial density. It follows them as they pass, passes with them. Does not the one that dies to the things and to the world know the imperative, not of becoming-nothing, but of becoming elemental, following the light beyond every direction, following the depth that deepens without end, following the reverberation of the vibrancy beyond one's situation and every situation in a world?

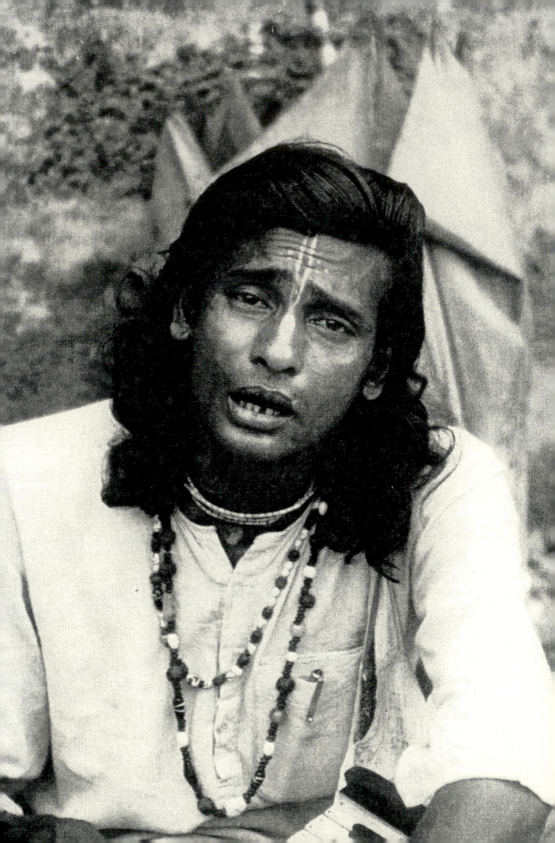

4

◆

The Body Postured
and Dissolute

We communicate with one another through signals, abstract entities, which have to be transmitted through the static and rumble of the world. Meanwhile, our bodies make contact with the fur seals, the spider monkeys, the agoutis, the hawks, the jaguars, the frogs, the rain, the leaves in the winds, the cliff path, the clouds, the flames, the earth, the remote stars. Making contact with them is not simply recording signals being randomly emitted by the friction and turbulence of things. We communicate with things by embracing them bodily. Our postures which are oriented upon them, converging our sensory surfaces on them, make contact with the sense—directions and directives—of things by being corporeally directed by them, by capturing their inner lines of position and movement. To make contact with things is to perceive the postures and gaits of things directing us. It is to discover oneself touched by alien hands, seen by alien eyes, heard by alien ears. The sensuality in us that diffuses as our performative mobilization and ego-control slackens makes contact with the materiality of things which induce transubstantiations in us. We communicate with one another in the exchange of information, but we make contact with inhuman things in embracing their forms and their matter. We also make contact with one another by contracting the other's form, and by transubstantiating our own material state.

THE POSTURE THAT RECOGNIZES AND IS RECOGNIZED

The *sensed* is not a momentary inextended impression or sequence of discrete impressions. A point of red, reduced to its here and now, is not the simplest component element in a visual phenomenon, because it is not visible. To be visible, it has to not be instantaneous or punctual; it has to endure and it has to spread its intensity across a certain expanse—and it has to contrast with its field, irradiate across a constellation of other colors, intensify other reds and stain other colors. A sound that does not resound is inaudible. The sounds we hear are chords, melodies, calls, cries, rattlings. We hear them in the midst of hum, rustling, rumble, static, clatter, or racket.

Sensing is not a passive reception of impressions on our sensitive surfaces. Sensing is a behavior, a movement, a prehension, a handling. To feel the tangible, the smooth, the sticky, or the bristly, the touching hand has to move across a substance with a certain pressure, a certain pacing and periodicity, a certain scope of movement. The look too, in order to see the red of the dress, has to focus, and move across its expanse with a certain pressure and scope and periodicity. One does not see the dull moss green of the leaves with the same movement of the look that makes the ardent red of the rose visible. It is in swaying with the melody, rocking with the rhythm, or being jarred by the clatter that we hear them.

Sensing does not simply record the fact of the red or the hard being there; it captures the *sense* of the red and of the hard. We recognize the sense of the lemon in seeing its opaque and homogenous color, its dull and rubbery surface, its homogenous and acrid odor. The sense or essence of the lemon is the way all that goes together and is sensed together. This sense is not an intelligible meaning, which could be captured in a concept. None of us have anything like an intelligible notion of what a lemon is; in fact, there is no concept of a lemon.

Traditional philosophy of mind had distinguished two operations involved in perceiving things: a passive registering of sensory impressions, and a collating or coordinating of them done by the central nervous system or by the mind. But the most elementary sensing already actively follows up patterns. Maurice Merleau-Ponty[1] has identified what perceives things as such, what comprehends the essence or the unity of things, to be what converges the sensory surfaces and movements: our body's postural schema.

The postural schema is the inner axis of a coordinated body directed on some object or objective. The postural schema of someone standing on a chair to unscrew the globe of a ceiling fixture and replace a burnt-out light bulb is continually being adjusted in response to the task; a movement of the hand induces a corresponding shifting of the trunk and tightening of the one leg, bending of the other. The actual posture then could not be the result of a program in the circuitry of the central nervous system, and the equilibrating and disequilibrating movements are not guided by a mental representation of the body's actual position. The postural schema is a dynamic gestalt, a structure such that any displacement of one part induces an ordered displacement throughout.

The postural schema is not only the unifying organization of the motor parts. Since every seeing of a color is done with a movement of the look, every feeling of a roughness or a resistance done with a movement of the hand, every hearing of a distinct sound done with a movement of the head that turns to center the ears upon it, the postural schema is also the unifying organizer of the sensory organs and surfaces. When, collapsed on the bed, one lets one's posture dissolve and legs and arms settle as the force of gravity determines, then finally one no longer senses things but an undifferentiated atmosphere or medium in which one is immersed. By converging our sensory surfaces on an objective, sensory properties consolidate and an intersensorial *thing* takes form.

A thing is not a whole assembled by the central nervous system out of separate sensory data, nor is it a conceptual term posited by the mind and used to interpret the data being recorded on the separate senses. The sense organ focused on a pattern is a segment of the whole interconnected mass of the sensory nervous system. What we pick up with the eyes is already sensed by the whole sensitive substance of our body. When we see the yellow, it already looks homogeneous or pulpy, hard or soft, dense or vaporous, it already registers on our taste and smell; anything that looks like brown sugar will not taste like a lemon. To see it better and to see it as a thing is to position oneself before it and converge one's sensory surfaces upon it. It is the postural schema that comprehends things. To recognize a lemon is not to conceive the idea of a lemon on the occasion of certain sensory impressions; it is to know how to approach such a thing, how to handle it, so that its distinctive way of filling and bulging out space, its distinctive way of concentrating color and density and sourness there becomes clear and distinct.

What makes sensory patterns be perceived as things are not outlines that circumscribe masses of sense-data but inner lines of force which position, and systematically move, a substance—something like *its* posture. To recognize a lemon in that lump of rubbery yellow there is to see the distinctive way this yellow occupies its space, holds and reflects the light, shades off in depth as its contours recede, to see how this yellow makes the inner substance surface, makes visible the pulpiness and the homogenous sour condensed there. One does not grasp something like the inner law or program, but one does catches onto the way the lemon will evolve before our sensory exploration. As a cloud passes over the sun and the light dims over it, the shift in its color will induce a corresponding shift in its tangible density. The lemon too is a dynamic gestalt; its features are in an active relation with the features of the environment and shifts in one feature induce corresponding shifts in others.

In the dim light of the end of the day we recognize our aunt coming down the sidewalk from a block or two away, at a distance too far to see the contours of her face or the hue of her complexion: we recognize the walk. Our acquaintances are those we stroll with, work with, look at things with. In perceiving them we do not look at their outlines and scrutinize their colors; our postures pick up their gait, their rhythms. We do not sit erect as the other lounges; our postures and the scope and periodicity of our gestures correspond.

The sense and recognizability of things too does not lie in conceptual categories in which we mentally place them but in their positions and orientations which our postures address. We recognize the pine on the hill by distinguishing not the distinctive color and shape of the needles but the upright and rigid stand; we recognize the willow by its loosely spread arms and the languid sweep of its branches. A fallen tree has lost its recognizability as a tree; it takes an act of imagination to visualize a tree in what we see as a log lying in a thicket. An armchair upside down looks like pieces of wood stuck in a mass of stuffing and fabric. In a crowded hospital room, when we find ourselves standing behind the head of the bed, the friend we look down upon is unrecognizable, his facial expressions look like muscular shiftings in a carnal mass and the smile, vexation, or query is no longer in them. We perceive the solemn erect stand of the court house posted on its pedestal of stairs, the military array of a phalanx of high-rises in a development project that is conquering the hills and the meadows of the bankrupt farmlands, the warm closure of the cottages nestled under the trees like brooding hens. We see the gun barrels of the smokestacks of the factory aimed at the heavens; we see the protective arch of the old country bridge under whose cool shade the ducks and the fish gather on hot days. We see the great rhythms with which the mountains and the pyramids of Teotihuacán rise through geological and sacred history to the sun and the moon. We see the sprint in the locust we contemplate on the twig, the plodding of the tortoise through the sprawling marsh, the languid stroll of the moth through the daisies dancing in the summer night.

SEEING ONESELF WITH ALIEN EYES

To assume a posture is to contract a "body image." As one sits at one's desk one has a sense of the visible shape with which one fills out a volume in the room; as one stretches one's legs under the table one has a sense of how their position looks. The more one's attention is absorbed in one's task and one's feeling in the orientation and rhythm of one's forces, the more determinate is this perception of the sides and outer contours of a thing one forms. This image is different from the patches of one's surfaces one is actually seeing and those one remembers. It fills out the outer aspect of one's body as it would be seen by someone viewing it from a distance sufficient to see the whole position or movement.

When the psychologist projects a videotape of people in silhouette walking across a landscape, one finds one can pick oneself out from among them by the gait. As one walks one cannot look at one's own gait, even in a mirror, for the observing eye interferes with one's natural gait and alters it. Since one can recognize it on the screen, one had while walking an immanent sense of the way one's gait looks from the outside. While maintaining one's momentum of preoccupied hurry through the streets, one gets a sense of the palpable thickness of one's limbs as they would be felt by others who would brush against one or crowd one. As we speak we have a sense of the sonority of our own voices as they would be heard by an ear not cupped against the teeth but at the distance we take from mouths to hear sounds spread in whole sentences. Although it is sometimes said that our own bodies have no perceived weight, when we move to be embraced and held by another and walk across the grass and climb the ladder we have a sense of the weight of our bodies as they would be felt by others and by the grass and the wood. What it is like to move in space capsules is hard to imagine.

What psychologists have improperly named the "body image" is not something projected by an act of imagination when one detaches one's perception from things; it emanates from the mobilized posture and thickens about its axes. The body in mobilizing into a posture situates the levels where other viewing positions lie and extends an "image" of itself as something visible, tangible, and audible in that space.

The vector of force I feel extending my leg also gives me a sense of what my leg extended under the table looks like; conversely, when I look at the outer aspect of my limbs and parts I get a sense of the inner lines of force and feeling in them. When I look at my own hand, I cannot see it as so much pulp molded over a bony framework; my eyes sense the orientation of dexterity extending it. When I look at myself in a mirror I feel my cigarette burning against the mirrored image of my fingers. When I am trying to pronounce phonemes or a foreign language or sing a new song, I listen to the sounds I emit and can thus pronounce them again, as though the audible pattern heard converts of itself into a motor diagram for my organs of vocalization. When the one hand touches the other the sense of a tangible mass hovers about the agile vector of sensibility of the touching organ, and in the felt mass of the touched hand a mobile vector of feeling stirs.

In the same way, when I look at the visible substance of another's hand, I sense there inner lines of force and feeling. I do not see these nor mentally diagram them but sense them directly with the dexterity of my own hand. My postural orientation directed on others is directed by them. Through just seeing someone seated on a stool, bench, or couch, my body finds spontaneously the posture corresponding to his as I go to join him. The posture of another is a diagram of vectors of vision and sensibility, and his look and gesture outline for me a position for my "body image" which my kinesthetic-coenesthetic forces settle in place. The visible figure the dance partner's limbs and parts extend before me is not observed and then interpreted in reversed projection. The infant that, at fifteen days, smiles at the sight of his mother's smile has not yet seen what his own face looks like and will never see the benevolence in the mind of the mother. He then does not set up in his mind an explicit relationship between the arc he sees in visual space, the muscular configuration in the body scheme of the mother, and the sentiment of benevolence produced in the mother's mind—and then between a sentiment of benevolence he produces in himself, a muscular innervation, and the resultant arc on his face as a visible surface. From the first the corporeal element that takes form doubles into motor schema and outward aspect, and the infant and his mother are superimposed in this reflexive circuit.

One's "body image" is not an image formed in the privacy of one's own imagination; its visible, tangible, audible shape is held in the gaze and touch of others. In sensing in and with their positions and moves the focusing of their vision and sensibility, the whole range of the visible, tangible, and audible shifts and refocuses, and one sees one's own visibility with their eyes, feels one's own tangibility with their hands, hears one's own voice with their ears.

Likewise, in perceiving the outer forms of things one captures in one's postural schema the inner lines of their tensions and orientations. And in contracting inner motor diagrams one quasi-perceives the visible, tangible, audible form of oneself turned to them. When we look at the sequoias we do not focus on them by circumscribing their outlines; the width of their towering trunks and the shapes of their sparse leaves drifting in the fog appear as the surfacing into visibility of an inner channel of upward thrust. We sense its force and measure its rise with the movement of our eyes and the upright axis of our body. We comprehend this uprightness of their life not with a concept-generating faculty of our mind but with the uprighting aspiration in our vertebrate organism they awaken. This postural axis emanates about itself a body image which is shaped not as the visual form our body would turn to a fellow human standing at normal human viewing-distance, but as our body looks to the sequoia. To see the weight of the rocks is to feel the diagram of a grip forming in our postural schema, and the weightless force in our arms now emanates about itself an immanent sense of the weight of our limbs the rock would feel as it struggles with our force. To see the magnesium flash-fires on the wind-caressed lake in the summer is to dance our eyes over it, and the look that cannot turn back to see itself emanates about itself a quasi-visual form of itself as seen by the vast eye of the lake. To listen to another is already to know how to myself pronounce what he or she says; the audible patterns he or she presents before me I capture on motor diagrams for my own speaking, and when I activate them in turn, the shaping and resonating of my breath through vocal chords and mouth emanates about itself an immanent sense of how my vocalizations sound to the other. As we hum while strolling across the fields and shout to the cliffs we hear how we sound to the murmuring meadows and to the great ear of the canyon.

It is one's own ligneous substance that perceives the sequoias; it is the hard and ferric substance of the bodybuilder's musculature that knows the inner essence of the steel; it is the blood pounding in his veins and the sweat glistening in sheets on his chest and back that know the flow of the rain and the coursing of the winds and the power of the sun. It is the clay of our own body, dust that shall return to dust, that knows the earth and knows itself as terrestrial; it is the liquid crystals of our eyes that are drawn to the stars as to brothers.

For our sentient bodies are not only vectors of force but substances. And transubstantiations are possible.

LUST FOR THE WORLD

How strange that the body's knowing that converges its sensitive surfaces upon things and contracts their postures turns to pursuit, penetration, detachment, dismemberment, dissection, that its knowledge is violent and cruel! The lines of the trees and the planes of the meadows, the levels the beams of sunlight set, and the contours of the moss-covered rocks and grass-covered earth that invite taking our bearings with our bared hands induce adjustment of our own body-axis in their midst. We may well enjoy this adjustment and the mobility it gives us and may wish to consolidate it by forceful means; we may wish to establish domination over our environment. But there is also a compulsion to break this adjustment and equilibrium and its contentment. The body that stands with the upward aspiration of the pines and the sequoias reaches out to break their limbs, that settles among the rocks with their mass and weight hurls them at one another, that bounds with the buoyancy of the wind-waved meadow lashes out at the flowers and butterflies as it strides. There is pleasure in knowledge, cruel pleasure in pursuit, penetration, detachment, dismemberment, and dissection. This pleasure is sensual, libidinal, Freud said.

Libidinal pleasure is not simply the psychic compensation the individual organism receives for obeying the imperative of species reproduction. Freud identified libidinal pleasure virtually at the beginning of life, in the slavering with which the infant drawing in the nourishment from the maternal breast deviates the organ-coupling into the production of a surface of surplus pleasure.

Of its own force, the organism repeats acts that no longer draw in sustenance, but produce pleasure. By an anaclitic deviation of the functional organ-coupling—any organ-coupling, mouth with maternal breast but also mouth with finger, mouth playing with the food, mouth playing with sounds, babbling, anus spreading the warmth of the excrement, hand not only holding but caressing and being caressed—pleasure-surfaces are produced. Infantile life discovers surfaces and the pleasures of surfaces, the pleasures of having surfaces, of being outside, of having been born. These surfaces function vitally to block the regressive death drive. This first infantile libido that extends an erotogenic surface is not a want or need, but a production. In this activity surplus energies are discharged; Freud, who saw in the discharges of genital orgasm the physiological model for all libidinal pleasures and all pleasures,[2] saw libidinal pleasure expressing the drive of an organism to return to the quiescence of the inorganic.

But the timeless, nonteleological libidinal drives repeat not only pleasurable states but also painful ones. The painful states when repeated generate sexual excitement. Sexual excitement does not show a simple drive for the release of tensions and quiescence; it reinstates tensions, even increases them. "It is easy to establish . . .," Freud writes, "that all comparatively intense affective processes, including even terrifying ones, spill over into sexuality."[3] Any relatively powerful emotion, even though it is of a distressing nature—Freud mentions intellectual strain, verbal disputes, wrestling with playmates, and railway travel—generates sexual excitement. "The compulsion to repeat presumably unpleasurable, repressed experience could therefore be understood as a permanent tendency on the part of the ego to resexualize its structure," Leo Bersani writes. "This would be done in the name of pleasure, just as any such shattering resexualization would also be resisted in the name of pleasure."[4]

We can then distinguish this libidinal excitement from the pleasure in the anaclitic deviation of an organ function, which the excitement would take all the way to a shattering of the psychophysiological organization. The drive in libidinal excitement in general, and its pleasure generated by the shattering of an established biological and physiological equilibrium and ego-control, is masochistic.

The focus and comprehensive integration of the postural schema would be, for Merleau-Ponty, the very consciousness of things, but the production of excitement in the shattering is also a broadening of consciousness. There are violent pleasures in the advance of knowledge. The cruelty of one's pleasure in things which one no longer couples onto but hunts down, exposes, severs, and sections, seeks in them a mirror of the shattering which pleasure pursues in oneself.

It is one thing to wish to exercise power over others, but why can we be sexually aroused by the suffering of others? Freud submits that the spectacle of pain in others produces a sense of that pain in oneself, which undermines one's control while generating sexual excitement. Such would be the pleasures of sadism where the masochistic identification with the suffering object can maintain one active with tensions that increase as the shattering that another suffers reverberates across one's intact organism.

Freud speaks of the precocious efflorescence of infantile sexual experiments and enterprises, a sensual life which is doomed to extinction because its wishes are incompatible with reality and with the inadequate stage of development which the child has reached. The capacity of the human psychophysiological system to resist or integrate, to "bind," the influx of sensation lags behind what its psychic identifications lead it to expose itself to. This would make the human child, born more helpless and maturing more slowly than the other mammals, particularly subject to the shattering of its structures of physiological equilibrium and ego-organization. The sexually precocious child fails to get all the love he or she wants, infantile sexual probings are unconsummated, he or she suffers sibling jealousy, fails to make babies himself or herself, suffers punishments from incomprehending parents, and suffers the increasing demands of socialization and culturation. The efflorescence of infantile sexuality, Freud writes, "comes to an end in the most distressing circumstances and to the accompaniment of the most painful feelings."[5] But the precociousness of the libidinal probings did not precede the distress and painful feelings; they rather fed one another.

Bersani, with Freud, still seeks to place libidinal excitement in the perspective of evolutionary progress. The supplement of exposure to shattering influxes of stimuli comes from the prematuration that engenders the behaviors of the human infant. An essential function of the human psyche is identification with figures of biological and sociocultural maturity in advance of itself. In the gap between established psychophysiological structures and ego-control functions which are shattered under the pressure of excess stimulation whether gratifying or unpleasurable, and another resistant or defensive equilibrium yet to be established, the influx of sensation that cannot yet be integrated spills over into libidinal excitement, which contains a drive to repeat and increase its pleasure. Libidinal excitement would then function as an incitant to shatter the equilibrium and ego-control one's biological and cognitive development had made possible. Libidinal excitement would be specific to humans—young animals try to mate, Bersani says, human juveniles seek libidinal excitement.[6] It would serve the transformation of the stages of their biological and physiological organization; it would be an inherited disposition resulting from an evolutionary conquest.

But is the pleasure of this excitement the pleasure of shattering established structures in the anticipation of more advanced, more integrated ones—or is it a pleasure just in suffering, in shattering established structures that made resistance, defense, and domination possible? To see a biological finality in sexual excitement is to suppose that it is in the anticipation of structures more integrated still, to be shattered in their turn, that sexual excitement could be not only aroused again, but increased. Yet Bersani concedes that the excitement itself is unmarked with regard to the types of structures involved. "We desire what nearly shatters us, and the shattering experience is, it would seem, *without any specific content.* . . . Sexuality manifests itself in a variety of sexual acts *and* in a variety of presumably nonsexual acts, but its constitutive *excitement* is the same in the loving copulation between two adults, the thrashing of a boundlessly submissive slave by his pitiless master, and the masturbation of the fetishist carried away by an ardently fondled silver slipper."[7] Libidinal excitement would be inherently solipsistic and masochistic, "a *jouissance* which isolates the human subject in a socially and epistemologically 'useless,' but infinitely seductive, repetition. . . . Sexuality would not be originally an exchange of intensities between individuals, but instead a condition of broken negotiations with the world, a condition in which others merely set off the self-shattering mechanisms of masochistic *jouissance.*"[8]

Yet Plato had seen in this "solipsistic" sexual excitement an exstasis that opens one to the outside, to the most remote dimensions of the universe. It is with worlds that we make love, Deleuze and Guattari write.[9]

What we call sex is many things. It is the innate reproductive organs and processes and drive. It is what Freud called libido—the swarming of nonteleological impulses seeking the pleasure unpleasure of excitement and which invest in representations. Psychoanalysis cannot measure libidinal impulses like forces and can only deduce them from an interpretation of representations—oneiric images, double-entendres, eruptions in the patent discourse of a stream of latent representations, actes manqués, obsessive and ritual acts, corporeal symptoms. The Freudian analysis of libido is a hermeneutics of the latent meaning of representations. What we call sex is also the theater of appearances, adornment, masquerade, simulation, and intrigue by which individuals make themselves attractive to one another, captivate and enslave one another—what Baudrillard has identified as seduction and distinguished from the sex of bared bodies and biological coupling.[10] What we call sex is also lust: the corporeal transformation itself—the shattering of the form that frees the substance, its transubstantiation, and the voluptuous pleasure of this transubstantiation. In addition to the biology of sex, in addition to the hermeneutics of libido psychoanalysis elaborates, in addition to the cultural anthropology of seduction Baudrillard calls for, we propose a material phenomenology of the corporeal transubstantiations experienced as lust.

Does not the direction of libidinal excitement which is imposed from the outside, and the shattering of the psychophysiological organization which is the frenzy of lust exposing one's carnal substance to that outside, contain a distinctive contact with the materiality of that outside? Far from being solipsistic, would not the masochistic pleasure desire to suffer transubstantiation from the outside and to open itself to the transubstantiations of the most remote things? Would the cruelty and violence lust unleashes, shattering the organization of things while shattering its own psychophysiological organization, be an incitement to these transubstantiations?

As the aroused body becomes orgasmic, it loses its postural integration; its limbs, dismembered, lie or roll freely, are moved with repetitive movements and convulsions. It stances and positions arrayed for objectives decompose; the hand that caresses moves aimlessly, not knowing what it is seeking, not gathering information, not moving itself intentionally but moved, agitated by the torments and pleasures that surface in the other. Lust muddies and makes turgid the light of thought, vaporizes its constructions, petrifies its ideas into obsessions and idols. Lust surges in the collapse of physiological equilibrium and ego-organization.

But this foundering does not prepare for the constitution of another set of structures of psychophysiological equilibrium and ego-organization. For in the collapse of postural organization and ego-control, there occurs a material *change of state*. The wanton frenzy surges in the flux from one material state to another; the tormenting pleasure flows with the transubstantiation.

Lust is the posture become dissolute, the bones turning into gum. The sinews and muscles lose their contractions to fill up with heat and susceptibility, the sweaty limbs quivering like exposed glands, the fingers spreading sweat and oils and secretions like aimless invertebrates. The torso loses its architectonic solidity to become a mass of ducts heavy with stagnant fluids and sludges. The eyes cloud and become wet and spongy, the mouth loosens the chain of its sentences, babbles, giggles, the tongue spreads its wet over the lips blotting out their muscular enervations. In the heat of this meltdown a mushrooming surge of sexual excitement tenses and hardens the body that gropes and grapples; then it collapses, melts, gelatinizes, runs in strange and impersonal pleasures. There is left the coursing of the trapped blood, the flush of heat, the spirit vaporizing in exhalations. Lust is the dissolute ecstasy by which the body's ligneous, ferric, coral state casts itself into a gelatinous, curdling, dissolving, liquefying, vaporizing, radioactive, solar and nocturnal state. The pleasures drift off and are lost, the body emptied of itself closes in like an infant to entrust itself to the anonymous forces that will reproduce its energies and its lusts.

The supreme pleasure we can know, Freud said, and the model for all pleasure, orgasmic pleasure, comes when an excess tension built up, confined, compacted is abruptly released; the pleasure consists in a passage into the contentment and quiescence of death. That is to confuse the pleasure itself with the torpor that will sink it into a sleep that will absorb the anonymous energies of the night. Is not orgasm instead the passage into the uncontainment and unrest of liquidity and vapor—pleasure in exudations, secretions, exhalations?

These convulsions and transubstantiations are not simply internal disintegrations of structures of psychophysiological organization and shatterings of ego-control; the excitement is provoked from the outside. The sensual experience of lust is a communication with what is most remote from the integrating, interpreting, decoding nature of the conscious ego; it is a communication with materiality in transubstantiation. It is provoked by the body of another divested of its socially coded uniforms, its body armor, its performative posture, dissolving in musks and sighs and torments of pleasure. It is provoked by the hard edges of reality radiating in twilight halos and perfumes, landscapes flowing into mists and languor, leaves incarnating into glands, rocks and sands liquefying and vaporizing, beams of sunlight caressing like fingers. The communication with the other that is in lust is not a communication with the idealized signals nor with the postures of things, but with their material states, a materiality freed from information and even from the formation into states—a materiality not holding its own forms, undergoing transubstantiations, suffering.

Lust finds idols and fetishes in human bodies and in the bodies of stallions and vipers, finds the philosopher's stone in the crepes and silks of garments and the plumes of exotic birds and those of cirrus clouds over the seas, petrified splendor in the powdered gestures of faces and arms and the iridescent flanks of sand dunes, time solidified in vaporous heaths, time sprinting in the flash fires of adamantine jewels.

To be sure, what we are here calling the surgings of lust occur in sex acts, that is, behaviors biologically programmed for reproduction, occur in the sociocultural theater of seduction, and occur in the directions fixed by libidinal investment in representations. To be sure, species reproduction lies ahead whenever a man approaches a woman with lust; the captivating appearances of individuals socioculturally made seductive with material and psychic adornments draw one closer to the lustful contact; the representations of self libidinally invested map out the directions in which the lustful contact may occur. To be sure, long hair and hard musculature are auxiliary features of individuals marked for genital intercourse, candlelight and wine represent grand-bourgeois distinction and *raffinement*, indolence and availability, leather represents hunters and outlaws, diamonds represent security forever. But lust cleaves to them differently. Encrusting one's body with stones and silver or steel, saturating one's skin with creams and lubricants till they glisten like mucous membrane, sinking into marble baths full of champagne bubbles or into the soft mud of rice paddies, feeling the grasses of the meadow or the algae tingling one's flesh like nerves, dissolving into perfumed air and into flickering twilight, lust seeks the transubstantiations of matter with a body in transubstantiation.

The one who plunges into the aimless night of lust descends into a Heraclitean cosmos, or rather chaos, not even ordered by the Law of Eternal Return of All Things, where earth becomes water and water becomes earth, air becomes fire and fire becomes air. Lust does not spring out of this miasma in order to return with messages and information to inform its postures and its images under the eyes of another or under the gaze of the sequoias or in the clasp of the steering wheel as it pulls us through the highways of the city. Lust dissipates and disseminates its forces, its fluids, its pleasures into the transubstantiating flesh of another, into the nervous fingers of sunlight and the landscapes flowing into mists and languor. The sleep it sinks into is not an inert death that would be its telos; it is the very reality of trust, the trust that the nocturnal movements of the planet and of the life on its hull will communicate the forces of their lust in return.

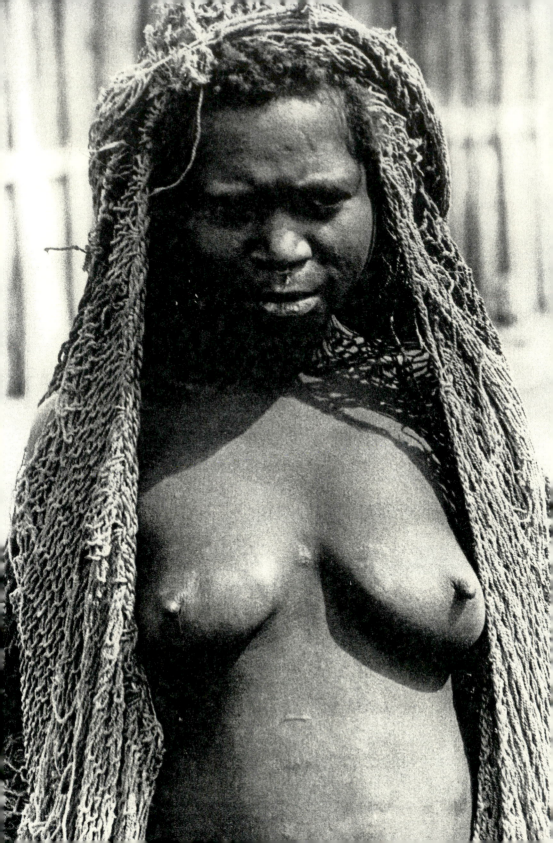

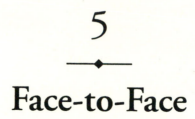

Face-to-Face

1. PHENOMENOLOGY OF THE FACE

THE OTHER

Face-to-face, we speak. What does a face do in facing? It does not only turn to me a surface, for my viewing, presenting contour and color; it does not only come within reach, exposing a tangible substance. In facing, another addresses me. In his or her face the other is other. By facing otherness itself takes up a stand over before me.

This distance of otherness opens up the interval of discourse. Across this distance, we speak.

The interval is a clearing for exposure. Things found elsewhere, things remote, absent, past, future, are going to be represented in that clearing. I shall be no longer surrounded by my own field of visions only, by the practical field geared in with my moves, where reality is what I take hold of and form with my eyes and my hands and retain in my concepts. Here the given takes form. For that is the marvel of language—just by our vibrating the air, gesturing in the emptiness, things get clear, reliefs and horizons get distinguished, a common world lights up. In the interval extended when the other takes a stand apart from me, and through the discourse that moves across that distance, reality is given.

Communication does not abolish the distance. In the word of greeting with which another addresses me and draws near, he or she sets before me his or her otherness. Each proposition and each response he or she makes to me marks again his or her stand apart. Without this distance, conversation and discourse, and the language that can sustain monologue and solitary inscription, would not be possible. Conversation moves in and presupposes, the world takes form in, the distance opened by alterity.

This distance opens in the difference between the surface another exposes to my view and the pressing want with which otherness seeks me out, between the substance the approach of another brings within reach and the intangible force with which I find myself touched and concerned. It opens in the difference between the surface and form my perception can take in and the indigence with which it solicits me, in the difference between the material which I can apprehend and the intrusion in that movement of material of which I am apprehensive. It opens in the difference between the one—another one, like me—I can represent to myself, as a counterpart of my own presence, and the other—other than me, other than what I can represent—who presents himself or herself. It opens in the difference between the other of whom I speak and the other to whom I speak.

This difference is felt in the pain of veracity.[1] In a moment of sincerity, I say to another what I have been saying about him. I present to him the concepts and formulations with which I had thought to circumscribe his presence and inform myself about who and what he is. Then I discover the irreducible difference between what I had been able to capture in my representation and interpret according to my own codes, and the other, who arises beyond, to contest, or to assent to, the image of him I have.

I can, to be sure, demand of the other that she tell her name and reveal her intentions. I aim to reduce her alien alterity, comprehend it with my own concepts, fit her presence into my own scheme of things. Yet even in assenting to my demands, the other shows her inalienable power to contest all my interpretations, and my interpretations of her words. She withdraws into her alterity in her very approach, and into the silence from which she came.

Speech is informative; in its movements things are not only linked up and ordered, but first take form. A given and common world takes form. And the other, whose move, whose facing, produced speech, also takes form in the interval it opened. But speech is also vocative and imperative. The first word of speech, a word of salutation, addresses me, calls upon me, appeals to me. Every informative and indicative proposition put to me also addresses me, calls up a me. I arise, out of the sensuous and pragmatic anonymity, in answer to this invocation. And speech does not only link up; it enjoins. It does not only inform and invoke; it orders. The proposition put to me by the other disturbs my order of things and representations, requires of them a justification. The word of the other contests me, has an imperative force.

Facing me, the other takes up a stand apart from me, and reveals himself or herself a stranger.[2] In his or her face there is eccentricity and exoticism. His or her alterity is not only the divergence of a difference—being in another place, coming from another moment—or of a dissimilarity—showing variations of properties on the ground of a recognized kinship. It is the distance of an abasement, a destitution and indigence that appeals to me. There is poverty and nakedness in the face of another. At the same time this distance is that of a height that contests and orders me. There is authority and majesty in the face of another.

THE DENUDING OF THE FACE

The other faces me with a glance, with a word, and with a gesture. There is nakedness in the eyes that look at me, powerlessness in the words that dissipate in the air, emptiness in the hands that gesture. Facing me, the other addresses an appeal to me.

What is more vulnerable, more naked than the eyes? The eyes do not shine, they speak—they appeal. Sartre had brought out all the strange force of the look that turns on me—it takes hold of me and fixes me in being. But it does so because it comes as a judgment. The objectification it effects is not a spreading out of my elusive subjectivity in the sensible field; I am already incarnate and sensible as a sensibility. It is a predicating of attributes of me, a contestation and a sanctioning. But the look of another judges me because it first makes demands on me, requires me and appeals to me. It is through the unassisted free mobility and the unprotected exposedness of the eyes that a nakedness rends the tissue of the material field. Things—bare walls, naked revolvers—are naked only by metaphor, when the naked demand of a look is refracted in them.[3] Even the erotic nudity, which appeals for the care and solicitude of kisses and caresses, derives from the extreme nakedness of a face. For only one who can face me can denude himself or herself wantonly.

With words the other faces. Language is not an instrument. In putting aside his or her arms and forces, in coming to me only in his or her words which hardly stir the air, which I can resist without doing anything at all—just by doing whatever I was doing—the other presents himself or herself in frailty and weakness. This way of coming, just to speak with me, calling to me to present myself, is the way of coming disarmed and disarming. This way of coming appeals to my presence, to my response and my resources.

The other faces me in a movement. The movements that face—gestures of his or her hands, dispositions of his or her posture—are not prehensions; they are movements that take hold of nothing, and address their emptiness to me. For a hand is not only an instrument, for seizing and taking. Hands are also organs for exploration; the hand that makes contact with the substantial and espouses it without taking possession of it is informed by it. The hand that makes contact with living substance, insatiably moving across it without removing anything from it, uncovering it without discovering anything, making contact with the spasms of alien life without learning anything, voluptuously luxuriating in its torment and tormented by its pleasure, enters into intimacy with another; the hand is also an organ for caressing. But when, in their supreme discretion, the hands take hold of nothing and form themselves with the emptiness, they speak. With such moves, empty-handed, the other solicits me.

It is true that the other who turns his or her face to me materializes before me. His or her detached mobility gives his or her visibility more abundance than even that of the solid things, fixed in their perspectives. Even mineral repletion, even granite and marble, seem to us to gain statuesque stability and monumentality when a face is formed in them. Yet the mobility of the face, if unconstrained by the connections of the surrounding forces, is also without effect on them; it does not move them but moves me. It moves me not by the cohesion of its forms but by its troubling vulnerability. The mobility of a face is not sovereignly arrayed with the force of its substance, but weighed down by it. Maturity brings it wrinkles, the traces in which the weight of its being is already the pressure of death.

The face materializes not under the manipulating hand, but under the eye and the touch that caresses. The caress is surface contact, contact with skin. The skin is neither functional like the protective cover over mechanisms nor significant like the tangible grain of wood that shows the structure of the interior. Skin is the surface which forms in wrinkles, the folds of weight and death. The touch that makes contact with the skin learns nothing but the distress of its own weight, the dying away of its pleasure and torment, the inconsequentiality of alien feeling. The touch learns only the impermanence of this impermeable substance—for the caresses push on to penetration, but, the erogenous zone extending like a Moebius strip, the kisses and coitions find only more skin.

The face with which the other presents his alterity to me is then neither a surface that reveals a depth, an aspect that exhibits an eidetic essence, a sign that transports one to an ideal sense-identity, or a phenomenon that makes a noumenon exist for-me. It is the trace of what does not present itself and is not representable, the pure passing of alterity, a denuding and dying that presses and solicits.

Facing me, the other calls upon me, and requires something of me. He or she requires that I respond, requires that I respond in my own name. Facing me, the other singles me out. He or she requires first that I be I, that I stand forth, present myself. Before the appeal of the other, I find that I always have something to say, something to offer, I continually surprise myself. I arise, out of the anonymity of sensible and utilitarian operations that go on in me, to find in myself inexhaustible resources. Before the face of another, I am always the rich one, I discover my existence as a superabundance.

THE SOVEREIGNTY THAT FACES

The appeal of the face is pressing and immediate. The other does not come first as an entity with being of its own, to then formulate its alterity. It is as other that the other speaks. The first word is the vocative move. This word is importunate and compelling; the destitution his or her face exhibits to me addresses me and calls unequivocally upon me because it orders me. His or her appeal solicits me because it contests me, it calls up the I because it summons it imperatively. His or her abasement in approaching me also situates him or her in height to order me;[4] if this way of being distant cannot be geometrically diagrammed, that is just what makes the nonspatial exteriority of alterity.

To speak is to be contested. To enter into language, to answer to the voice of another, is to expose oneself to contestation. To recognize his call and his question is already to recognize his rights over me, his right to question me. It is already to recognize the ascendancy of alterity, the sway of the move that faces, the authority of the face.

I can, to be sure, by doing nothing, by refusing to budge from my silence, refuse to recognize the other, deny his right to question me. I can in what I say contest her in my turn, adjudicate the claims she makes on me, question her right to judge me. But these responses are possible only because alterity already faces, and speaks imperatively. Every putting of him in his place, every reification or objectification of alterity, determination, deduction or induction of her nature and powers, already every representation of his or her presence, is already a response made to his or her passing.

The other's facing comes as a disturbance of order. The order of things—which is first their spatial array about my position, their temporal flow through my zone of presence, their dynamic coupling onto my powers, the gradations of their appropriation by me—the order through which my freedom arises, is troubled from without. Not by a foreign element, which could eventually be fitted into the system of things, or, if not, serve as the occasion for a new, more encompassing order. The move of alterity is an intrusion, a contestation. It does not merely compete with me for the things I have made exist for myself; that is what the other does when he or she marshals his or her forces counter to mine, rather than expose his or her face to me. The move of alterity commands the very ordering by which my freedom takes power. When otherness faces me, it orders me to reorient all the things that exist for me so as to make them common—objective, givens or gifts.

The voice of alterity orders me to the core, in the nucleus of the ego in me. It dislodges the selfness by which my life vibrated upon itself in the contentment of sensible pleasure and the assimilation of my surroundings. It compellingly summons an I to respond, summons up an essentially responsible ego, an ego constituted in the recurrence of responsibility.

2. THE FACTS OF RESPONSIBILITY

The otherness of the other is envisaged and not viewed, responded to and not represented. The encounter with the other is a being affected by him or her— one's own resources and substance being drawn off by him or her, one's labors giving to him or her. To recognize the other is not to re-cognize another "one" nor to identify alterity; it is to recognize not the form and distinctive aspects of the face, but the force—a vocative and imperative, and not a causal, nor an indicative and informative, force—of the facing. It is to acknowledge a claim; it is to answer to his or her appeal and respond to his or her order. It is not to act on him or with him, but to be responsive, with one's being exposed, with full arms and not with words only. The relationship with alterity is responsibility before the other and for the other.

Responsibility constitutes the subjectivity that has the form of the I. To find oneself faced with another is first to hear a summons to arise, to present one-self. The I that answers arises out of the anonymity of the sensibility that savors the materiality of the sensible elements, that is immersed in the sustaining and nourishing medium of the world. One puts oneself forth in expressive moves, by which one exposes oneself to the other—not in order to achieve recognition for oneself and to consolidate oneself in being, but in order to answer for the wants of the other and order oneself according to his or her imperatives. Responsibility is not only realized in leaving to the other one's concepts or one's catch, one's properties, one's possessions; from the first one makes oneself available, one's position and resources sustained by the nourishing medium of the elemental. The fundamental figure of responsibility is not the citizen-legislator, but, Levinas says, maternity.[5]

It is before the other for the other that I am responsible. To be responsible is to put oneself in the place of another, not in order to observe oneself from without, and not in order to displace him or her or take from him or her his or her own tasks and destiny, but in order to supply for his wants, to be a support for her indigence, to bear the burden of his or her passing. It is to be answerable for her need and nakedness, and for the move with which he requires and denudes himself, for its imperative urgency, for his or her exactions and failings. It is to be answerable before the other in his or her alterity and not in his or her empirical dissimilarity or numerical difference. Responsible before all the others for all the others, held accountable for the deeds and misdeeds of others, for the very responsibilities of others, the I exists, Levinas says, in the figure of a hostage.[6]

How far does responsibility extend? It is already in effect. Its scope is not comprehended at once by a concept; it is responsibility that recognizes responsibility. The more one undertakes to bear the burden of existence, the greater are the demands put on one; the more one justifies oneself, the more extensive one finds the contestation put on one. Responsibilities increase in the measure that they are taken up. They are incumbent in this unterminatedness. The very alterity of the other, ever more unassimilated and uncomprehended, is in this unfulfilled, unfinished extension of his or her requisition, this infinition.

Responsibility does not originate in, and is not measured by, a commitment the subject would have imposed upon itself. It is a fact, laid on and not posited by subjectivity. I am not only answerable for what I initiated in a project of my will. (The courts measure no penalty for the genetic defect I passed on to my child, but to be a parent is to supply for his disability with my own strengths.) I am answerable for the existence in which I find myself; responsibility is a bond between my present and what came to pass before it. To be responsible is always to have to answer for a situation that was in place before I came on the scene.

Heidegger saw at the bottom of conscience and the need to justify oneself that want or failing with regard to oneself, the existential guilt, which is the situation of a being that has to take over powers of existence it has not itself constituted—the situation of a being that has been born.[7] This shortfall with regard to one's own existence would be at the bottom of the guilt of deeds and omissions that produce deprivations in the world and in the existence of others. The responsible one has to take over an existence that has been born; its responsibility would express the bond between its presence and its having come to pass, its birth. I envision acts that would be my own by envisioning the range of possibilities my oncoming death circumscribed before me, and I make my acts my own by answering for them; in doing so I take hold of the time that is my own—the span from my birth to my death.

For Levinas responsibility is not having to answer for my being on the scene, but having to answer for the post at which I was stationed, in a situation made by others. Responsibility links the actual time of my action with another time, the time of others. Each time the I finds itself, faced by another, it finds itself present to answer for a move of alterity that has already come to pass. The present in which my action is born finds itself bound to answer for a time before it was born, and for what came to pass before I was born.

I am responsible for developments in which I find myself, and which have a momentum by which they go on beyond what I can carry out or steer. Responsibility cannot be limited to the measure of what I was able to foresee and willed. My force of initiative has force only inasmuch as it espouses things that have a force of their own. Is not taking oneself to be responsible for what will happen to our affairs after we are no longer there what makes up the seriousness of any responsibility we recognize? My death will mark the limit of my force without limiting my responsibility. By responsibility, the time which subjectivity makes its own opens upon the time of the others. It is in the presence of the others, and not before the nothingness to come of its death, or the nothingness that came to pass in its birth, that subjectivity extends in responsibility.

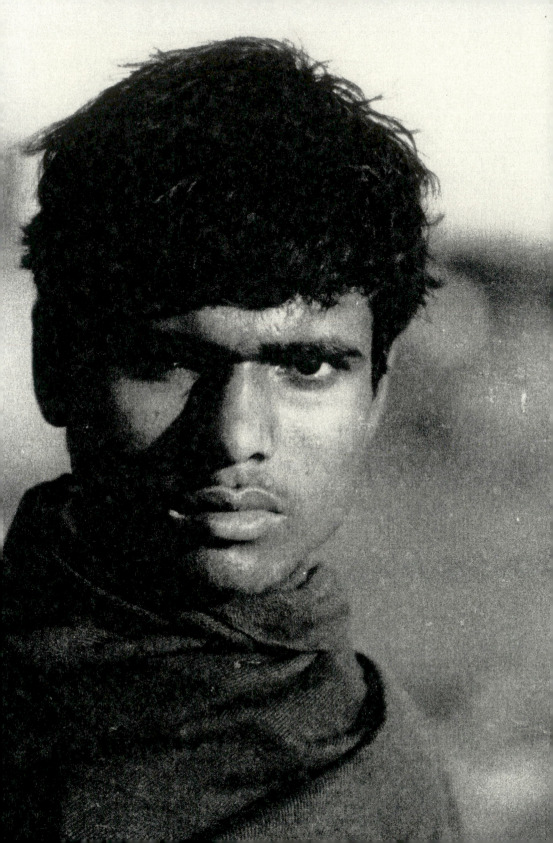

6

◆

Sensuality and Sensitivity

To sense something is to catch on to the sense of something, its direction, orientation, or meaning. Sensibility is sense-perception, apprehension of sense. But to sense something is also to be sensitive to something, to be concerned by it, affected by it. It is to be pleased, gratified, contented, and exhilarated, or to be pained, afflicted, and wounded, by something. A sentient subject does not innocently array object-forms about itself; it is not only oriented in free space by their sense, it is subject to them, to their brutality and their sustentation.

The sensibility that is in our nervous circuitry was implausibly conceived as a passivity of the mind upon which the physical action of the material world taps out impressions, which a free and spontaneous understanding can then take as signs, forming, relating, and positing referents for them. Is receptivity passivity? Is there in it a synoptic assembling of the multiplicity of sense data? Is there in it an intentional orientation? But is the sensuous element really a multiplicity of discrete impressions? Is the affective sensitivity but a side-effect of sensibility, a factor of confusion and indistinctness in sense perception? Is there opposition between sensibility and responsibility—between the sensibility for sensible things and the sentiment of respect, which Kant called the receptivity of the spontaneity of the mind, the sensibility of the faculty of understanding? Were the metaphysical correlates of matter and form, activity and passivity, really imposed on the classical philosophy of mind by analysis of the phenomenon of sensibility?

There is a movement in sensibility. In the receptivity for sense, the capacity to catch on to the orientation and potentialities of things, Martin Heidegger has seen the propulsion that makes our being exist, that is, cast itself out toward entities exterior to itself, and cast itself beyond them to take in the context in which they could move. Our existence is sensitive; our sensibility moves with the movement of existence, ex-ists. The given beings make an impression on us because the active, self-propelling thrust of our being makes contact with them, and beyond where and how they are actually to their possible positions and employment, their futures. What we sense when we sense the solidity of the seat is neither a coagulation of chromatic and tactile impressions nor an idea, an ideal object, associated with them; it is a possibility. Sense-perception is in fact an apprehension of the forces of things, the possibilities things are, an anticipation of the future of the environment, a clairvoyance.

Our eyes focus, follow the light, circumnavigate the contours, sweep across the colored and shadowed expanses; our hands stroke the grain and the textures; our tongues circulate the brandy in our mouths; our postures center our sensory surfaces on things; our legs and torsos bear our movements. The existential movement in perception animates our bodies.

But the propulsive force by which our existence casts itself perceptively into the environment is oriented by the layout of things. There is subjection to the outlying environment in the sensibility.[1] Our emotions disclose to us, in us, how the things we envisage matter to us; our affective disposition, our moods, reveal how the layout as a whole besets us. It is not with their "primary properties," their contours, but also not with their forces, their instrumental potentialities, that the things first affect us; they trouble us by being there. Affectivity, far from being just a subjective factor of confusion and immanence in the mind, is a revelation of the environment, a revelation of its being. The environment is not only a layout of contours whose orientation, sense, and future we envision; in our affectivity the fact of their being there of themselves is imposed on us. We find ourselves exposed not merely to the phosphorescent appearances of things that are closed in themselves but to the incontrovertible plenum of their being, to all the infinity of the condensation with which their being has replaced and excluded nothingness. It is in itself that our being knows the being of the most remote things, of the whole environment. Heidegger says that while our existence distances itself from, and posits apart (*entfernt*), the forms and appearances of things through sensibility, our being is afflicted from the start with the pressure, the gravity, of the being of those exterior things.[2] Our own being is exposed to the being of the most alien and remote things from the start, exposed to the dimensions of remoteness in which beings can be exterior; the weight of the being of the environment presses down on us. In fact the ecstatic thrust of our existence by which we cast ourselves beyond their actual forms and positions to their possibilities is not really a free-floating domination over them; it is a continual effort to escape the burden of their being which oppresses our being from the start.[3]

These two sides to our original contact with the environment—projection into it and subjection to it, delineating a line of sense in it and being beset with the fact of its being—Heidegger sought to make intelligible, in their juxtaposition in our sensibility, by understanding them as dimensions of the movement of time, the inner time of our existence.[4] Our presence is realized as an ecstatic transport from the state of being disposed by the environment to the synthetic grasp of its possibilities, a transport conjoining projective comprehension with affective subjection, sensibility with susceptibility, a transport of what has come to pass in us to what is to come to us, an existential transport of the being we have been given to our potentiality for being otherwise.

But this transport itself, Heidegger will show, is nothing else than the active realization of the subjection of one's being to nothingness, which is our vulnerability or our mortality.[5] The propulsion of the sensibility beyond the given to the possible, beyond the present to the imminent, beyond the entity into the space of the world, is in fact a projection into nothingness. The possibility that the sensibility grasps in the exterior is not simply a representation, an advance presentation of another format of the sensible surfaces drawn by the power of the mind to vary their actual appearances. It is also not simply the arrangement of them that is not yet there and which the mind perceives in advance. Neither the calculative skills of the mind nor its recombinatory imagination produces the real possible. The possibilities are the future of things, but a future which is not ineluctable, which is possibly impossible. The sensibility that reaches for the sense of things makes contact with impossibility in them.

When the perception that reached for the possible falls into the impossible, it reaches for adjacent possibilities in the environment. But the impossibility that lurks in any of them lurks in all; the being of the whole environment which besets our being is but a possible being, and possibly impossible. The weight and force of the world's being that presses down on our being is also the imminence and ineluctability of nothingness in which the contingent world is suspended, and which we sense in the mortal lucidity of our anxiety. The world that solicits us with its possibilities and promises, and that incites our existence to continually project itself out toward it, draws by withdrawing into its own being and into the imminent nothingness that does not cease to threaten its irremediable contingency.

It is this mortal lucidity of our anxiety that makes our existence perceptive, our sensibility clairvoyant. At the bottom of our concern for the possible beings there is a sense of being singled out by the nothingness that approaches of itself, that closes in, that touches us already. It is because we are first stricken with the void, haunted by the death everywhere lurking in the interstices of the world, affected by its nothingness, that we are touched, affected by, stabilized and steered by things, that the things have sense for us. They have sense and affect us not as material nor as forms, but as means, supporting gear or obstacles and snares in the way of our movements into the environment. It is with one and the same movement that our being projects itself into the open clearing of a world and into the emptiness of impossibility, the void of the definitive and irreversible abyss of death. Being-in-the-world and Being-unto-death are one and the same.

For Heidegger it is thus because we are exposed to nothingness that is exterior to all being that we are exposed to exterior beings. For Emmanuel Levinas sensibility is exposure not to nothingness but to alterity. And for him otherness is not decomposable into being and nothingness; possibility is not decomposable into actuality and the impossibility that threatens it.

Levinas's phenomenological exposition shows that prior to the anxious taking hold on things which for Heidegger makes our sensibility practical from the first, there is the contact with the sensuous medium, there is sensuality.[6] We find things, we find ourselves, in the light, in air, on terra firma, in color, in a resonant zone. Through sensuality we find ourselves steeped in a depth before we confront surfaces and envision the profiles of objects. Sensibility opens us not upon empty space, but upon an extension without determinate frontiers, a plenum of free-floating qualities without substrates or enclosures, upon luminosity, elasticity, vibrancy, savor. The sensuous element—light, chromatic condensation and rarefaction, tonality, solidity, redolence—is not given as a multiplicity that has to be collected or as data that have to be identified, but as a medium without profiles, without surfaces, without contours, a depth, an *apeiron*. We find ourselves in it, in light, in the elemental, buoyed up, sustained by it. Life lives on sensation; the sensuous elemental is sustenance, end, goodness of being we enjoy before any practical intention arises to locate means for our pursuits.

Sensuality is not intentionality, is not a movement aiming at something exterior, transcendent, that objectifies; it is not identification of a diversity with an eidos, an ideal identity term; is not imposition of form or attribution of meaning. Steeped in the elemental, contented with the plenum, its movement is that of enjoyment.[7] The enjoyment is the vibrancy and excess of our openness upon the elements, which delineates the movement of involution and ipseity: being sensual, one enjoys the light, the color, the solidity, the spring, the monsoon, and one enjoys one's enjoyment. The most elementary egoism in sensitive flesh is this eddy of enjoyment reiterated; the first ego is a pleasure.

Sensuality is vulnerable and mortal from the start. But this susceptibility inseverable from sensibility is not the vertiginous sense of the contingency of all being, the imminence of nothingness threatening one in all beings one touches. The sense of the contingency of the sensible medium, a flux or chaos without law or necessity, supported by nothing behind its appearing—for the things will be formed in it, out of it—is not to be identified with an intuition into the nothingness in which all being would be perilously adrift, and which could be foreseen as a real possibility just beyond the thin screen of the actual being. The contingency of the sensuous element is in the very fullness and abundance of the present, which plugs up the horizons, the future. Coming from nowhere, going nowhere, it is there by incessant oncoming. It is not there as though grudgingly parcelled out by the malevolence of nothingness, but as gratuity and grace. Fortuity and goodness of the light, the vibrant colors, the radiance of tones, the liquidity of the swelling forces! Yet there is in sensuality a sense of vulnerability, not made of anxiety over the imminence of nothingness but of the liability of being wounded and rent and pained by the force and substantiality of the sensuous element. In pain one is backed up into oneself, mired in oneself, in-oneself, materialized; pain announces the end of sensibility not through a conversion into nothingness, annihilation, but at the limit of prostration, conversion into passivity, materialization. In savoring the materiality of things sensibility has the taste of its own mortality. It is in the materiality of being and not in its inconsistency, its being already undermined by the imminence of nothingness, that our death already touches us.

If Heidegger finds, subtending the capacity to be affected by the impact of beings, an exposure to or a projection into nothingness, it is because he conceives of sensibility as an outbreak of freedom from the start, an intentionality or transcendence. There is sensibility for beings and presence to being when our existence finds itself exposed to nothingness, or finds itself in a clearing or free space. He conceives of our existence being open as being an openness. Its first model is the hand that has leeway to move; he conceives of sensibility as handling things. The hand that reaches out for possibilities in things risks impotence. It is by being a possible menace that a means is an implement. It is by being a possible impasse and snare that the direction or orientation of a thing makes sense.

Levinas takes instead finding oneself in the light, in vibrancy and plenitude, as a primary model of what happens when life becomes a lucidity. He finds in the tremor of sensation not an exhilaration and ecstacy out of being, but an enjoyment, an intensity and an involution. For Heidegger things are implements grasped by their forms—not shapes outlined by a contemplative eye, but interlocking contours relaying and orienting a body force on the move. For Levinas, things are first substances, contained within their contours which lend themselves to being detached, moved, and destined for enjoyment. Things are drawn from the sustaining medium, and things grasped instrumentally revert to an elemental presence. One grasps the hammer to pound in the nail, but in the hammering the hammer becomes a substance sustaining the rhythm of the hand that enjoys hammering. The contours of things are not limits beset by nothingness, but delineations of alterity, reliefs in the elemental plenum.

Levinas's extended analysis of sensibility contains the bold and strange thesis that the exposure and subjection to beings is itself subtended by an exposedness and subjection to alterity.[8] He reverses the Kantian position; for him responsibility, sensitivity to others, does not conflict with and mortify sensibility for mundane beings, but makes it possible.

Heidegger already had located responsibility not in one suprasensorial faculty, the rational faculty, but in the sensible structure of our existence. Responsibility is not a receptivity for an ideal order, an order of the ought over and beyond what is. For Heidegger being is the law; it is being that orders and ordains. His *Introduction to Metaphysics*[9] initiated a diagnosis of the period when metaphysics extended its sway over all Western culture, determining the meaning of being by separating being from, and opposing it to becoming, appearing, thought, and the ought. For us being is the given, the actual, the facts, over against what ought to be. Heidegger repudiates this opposition; for him it is being that binds us, obligates us, is the law and the destiny. He will show this by showing that being in us is not just what is coextensive with us as the matter of our movements or the actuality of our acts. Between us and our being, there is not coinciding but relationship: in us our own being is a matter of concern. For us to exist is to relate to our being; we consider our being here, question it, are troubled, afflicted by it, wearied with our own being. But our being is not an object we envision; it affects us, weighs on us, afflicts us. Our affectivity is a sense of our responsibility for our own being. We do not engender our being; it is given to us, laid upon us; we are burdened with it, and have to bear it. We do not exist, simply; we have to be. Being in us is an imperative: we are bound to be. Socrates too felt that, when he castigated suicide as recreancy and desertion. The imperative is first an imperative to exist—in order to answer for existence.

This way we have to be related to our own being such that it affects us, weighs on us, is at the origin of the existential option being made between existing inauthentically, that is, anonymously, or authentically, that is, on our own. The primary awareness of our being is an effort to take a distance from it, to evade the burden of having our being as our own, of having to be on our own. Feelings contracted from others, passed on to others, perceptions equivalent to and interchangeable with those of any other, thoughts which conceive but the general format of the layout about one, sentences formulated such that they can be passed on to anyone—make up the rigorous and consistent enterprise of evasiveness in the face of the being that is one's own to be. Evasiveness in the face of one's own being is an evasiveness in the face of one's own time. It makes us live each day as it comes, making it a reinstatement of the day that passed, expecting always another day to take the place of the one that is passing; it makes us live out time as an indefinite succession of nows, of manageable units, workaday workdays. What makes us so continuously and consistently evasive with regard to the being that is our own to be is the fear of the anxiety that has never ceased to be felt over the nonbeing that is our own to become.

Responsible being originates at the far end of anxiety. The anxiety that rehearses dying, that anticipates the limits of what is possible for me, casts itself over and takes over the full range of what is possible for me, unto the last limits of impossibility. The anxiety that anticipates the nothingness that is to come for me delivers over to me the full range of all that is mine to become. One becomes responsible in anxiety.

It is one's own being that is imperative; the being that is given to me is a destination to a potentiality for being which my actual being engenders, and a destination to the nonbeing that is to come for me.[10] The imperative is an imperative not for the universal and the necessary, but for the singular; it is the imperative that my singular potentiality for being come to be. At the same time, however—and this is the central hinge forged in Heidegger's existential ontology—the being in me that I appropriate is being, being generally. In my own being the being of the world, universal being, presses upon me. I cannot answer for my own being without undertaking to answer for the being of all that is. That is why I am a pulse of care in the universe, not only anxious for my own exposed, vulnerable, mortal existence, but concerned for the world, for all that is. For Heidegger it is this being afflicted with, being concerned for, the contingent being of a world, and not merely anxiety over my own subsistence, that makes my existence practical. Responsibility is finding in the forces of my own existence the wherewith with which to come to the assistance of universal being, threatened throughout with nothingness. Responsibility is, he says in his late writings, to shelter the most remote things, earth, heavens, harbingers of the immortal, in my own mortal existence.

Responsibility is then not measured by authorship; it is not just the will or the project to answer for what originated in one's own existence. It takes over and answers for a situation one did not initiate; it is answering for what one did bring about, for what came to pass before one was born, for the deeds and failings of others. And responsibility answers already for the sequence of occurrences that extend beyond the force of one's own that steered them, answers already for what will come to pass when one will no longer be there.

Responsibility is coextensive with our sensibility; in our sensibility we are exposed to the outside, to the world's being, in such a way that we are bound to answer for it. A world is not just a spectacle spread before us but a burden we are entrusted with. What opens us to the exterior, what makes us exist, be a sensibility, is exteriority, which approaches of itself, and touches us, affects us, afflicts us. For Heidegger this exteriority is what is exterior to our being and to all being: nothingness or death. The approach of this exteriority is also what casts us back upon our own being and upon all being, and makes existing for us a response to the nothingness and a responsibility for being.

For Levinas, it is not the encounter with nothingness that could make us take on our own being and answer for all being; it is alterity. Alterity is not nothingness, which could only be as the nihilation of being. It is not ideality, self-sufficient and absolute in its immobile present. Alterity is what is positive enough to appeal to being, and separate enough from it to imperatively order it. This kind of alterity Levinas locates neither in the death that summons all that lives, nor in the ideality of law, without executive force, but in the face of another. For the face is not the surface of another being. In his face, by facing, the other takes a stand; otherness itself appeals to us and contests us.

In *Totality and Infinity* Levinas has worked out the phenomenological analysis of facing in such a way as to show that the perception of the face of another is a responsibility.[11] In turning to face me, the other signals me; his face, his expression, his word, is not only indicative, informative, but also vocative and imperative. She faces me with her eyes, unmasked, exposed, turns the primary nakedness of the eyes to me; she faces me with a gesture of her hand, taking nothing, empty-handed; she faces me with a word, which is not an instrument, an arm, which is the way to come disarmed and disarming. To recognize his or her move in facing is to recognize an appeal addressed to me, that calls upon my resources, and first calls upon me, calls upon me to stand forth as I. And he or she appeals imperatively. To recognize his or her voice is to recognize his or her rights over me, his or her right to make demands on me and to contest me, his or her right to demand that I answer for my existence.

There are then two kinds of sensibility: a sensibility for the elements and things of a world, sensuality, which is appropriation and self-appropriation, and a sensibility for the face of another, which is expropriation and responsibility. But in *Otherwise than Being*, Levinas sets out to show that the space in which the sensuous material is laid out is already extended by the sense of alterity which takes form and becomes a phenomenon in the face of another.[12] This thesis involves the idea, already found in Heidegger, that before the beings of the outside world are set forth for me, they are possessed by others; that the material world is "human" even before it is a nourishing medium. That its elements are "objective" or "intersubjective," elements in themselves or open to others, before they are goods for me.

It is true that already in Husserl and in Heidegger the lateral relationship with others, as other points of view, or as other sites where being is exhibited, entered into the constitution of universal space. But Levinas advances two innovations. First, he thinks that the relationship with the other does not only enter at the point where my perceptual field, already extended by my own intentional perception or by the reach of my utilitarian operations, is fitted into impersonal universal extension; for him spatial distance is not extended by a sense of nothingness but by a sense of alterity. Secondly, the relationship with alterity can have this role because the relationship with the other is not, as in Husserl, perceptual, or, as in Heidegger, pragmatic, but ethical. There is then a difference of levels; the argument is not that the other is the first object of perception, or the first instrument with which one could get one's bearings in a field of things. It is that what institutes the first *here*, what constitutes my existence as here, is not the power to keep objects at a distance, but is the pain of being afflicted with the demands of the other.

For Heidegger what subtends the sense of space is the sense of nothingness; the space of the world is the very abyss of death. This is because Heidegger takes being to be presence, *ens* to be *prae-ens*, and presence to be dis-stancing distance. The *Entfernung* which realizes presence is situating at a distance, and Heidegger took the sense of distance and exposure to contain a sense of nothingness in general and in itself. In boredom and in anxiety nothingness nihilates; in antagonism, rebuke, failure, prohibition, privation nothingness nihilates— in all distance, including all separateness by which things take their stand about us, nothingness nihilates.

For Levinas what extends space is not the nothingness that separates and frees the entities of a world to be as they are where they are; it is contact, contact with what is other and withdraws in the midst of the contact. He first worked out the notion on the example of the neighbor whose proximity, whose nearness, consists in his touching us, affecting us, while remaining uncomprehended, unassimilable by us. In this move, a neighbor is other, shows himself as other. This occurs when the other faces us, that is, appeals to us, contests us.

The contact does not only reveal the proximity of the other; it determines the *here*, determines the one contacted as here. Being here, being a here in being, supposes in our substance not only a capacity to be oriented or disposed by the exterior but a susceptibility to being affected, altered—sustained and wounded. To be here is to be exposed to the other, exposed to pain.

Quite early Levinas studied the immanence of pain. To be pained is to feel one's own substance, as a passive affliction, in the torment of wanting to escape oneself. For to escape pain would be to be able to transcend it toward the world, or to be able to retreat behind it and objectify it. The inability to flee or retreat, the being mired in oneself, is the suffering of pain.

Later Levinas was to find this inner diagram of pain in the contact with the other. The approach of the other who faces, afflicting one with his exigencies and exactions, throws one back upon oneself. One is unable to establish distance by rendering present to oneself, representing to oneself, what afflicts one so pressingly. One is unable to retreat from the demand by apprehending or comprehending it, setting it before oneself by one's own initiative as though it emanated out of oneself. One finds oneself forced back into the resources of one's own being by the exaction put on oneself. This being backed up into oneself, this having to bear the burden and affliction of the other's wants and failings without being able to find anyone to take one's place, this being held to one's post, repeats, in the structure of the one being approached by alterity, the inner diagram of pain. Thus the *here* is fixed. To find oneself somewhere is to be exposed, not to emptiness and nothingness, but to suffer appeals made on one's substance and contestations made of one's stand.

The recognition of the imperative in the face of another is not an abstract and intellectual respect for the pure form of the law which the other would instantiate on the diagram of his moves; it is the recognition of a claim put on my substance and my life, the injunction to answer for the destitution of others with one's own bread and, a hostage, to give one's life in sacrifice. The other's wants are first material; they make claims on my own sustenance, made wholly of the substance of the sensuous element. It is not only some surplus of my possessions that is contested by his imperative need, but my appropriative life by which I appropriate myself. Responsibility is serious when it is not only my surplus that is affected but all that sustains my life and my very occupancy of this post.

To have to answer to the other is to have to answer for what I did not initiate and for his or her wants and failings and even for his or her approach that puts me in question. It is this position that is constitutive of my being here, and of my being vulnerable to being wounded by entities. The exactions put on me by others make me liable to death—not by taking away the ground under my feet and casting me into the void but by exposing me to the obduracies and lacks of material things. It is not in being delivered over to nothingness, it is first in being delivered over to beings, having to count only on their sustenance, that I am mortal. To this mortality I am delivered by the exactions of alterity; from the first a claim is put on my life, on my life living on the enjoyment of life.

Thus we find Levinas's texts taking on some of the pathos of the Kantian moral philosophy, for which the inclination to obey the moral imperative is always received as a humiliation and a pain by the sensuous nature of man. But in Levinas this pain is not only the intellectual pain of feeling negated and frustrated, even when the moral order is carried out by the executive forces of life; it is the pain of substantial wounding and of sacrifice demanded of life. For it is in depriving oneself to answer for the hunger of those who have no claim on one but their hunger, and in sacrificing oneself to answer to others for what one did not do, that responsibility is serious.

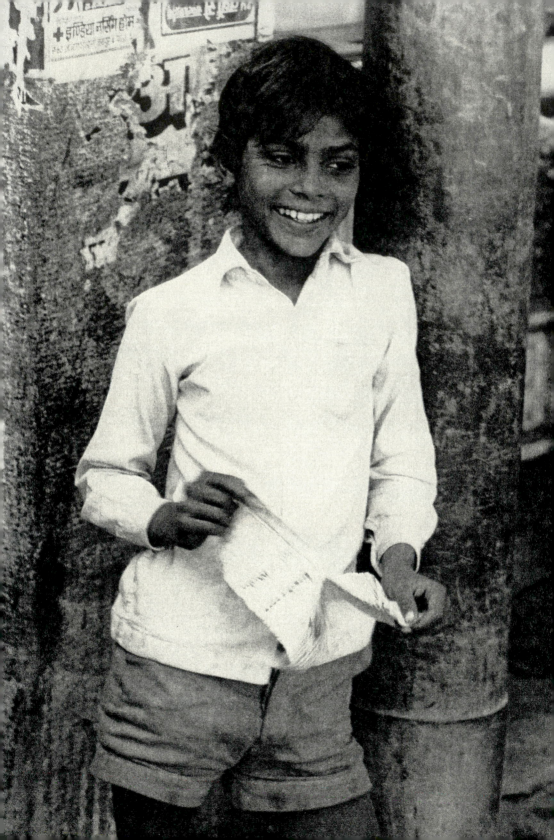

7

◆

What Is Passed Over in Communication

Thinking about what one sees, formulating it, which produces truth out of meaningful relations with the environment about one, produces insignificance. Not only in being recalled in the wrong experience, in the wrong situation— just in being recalled. In communicating what one sees, one loses sight of it. Not by communicating it at the wrong time, in the wrong context; its very truth, in being spoken to another, empties out.

Insight is proclaimed in an "Aha!" It is then formulated in a distinctive utterance that aims to record just this insight: "I see that S is p." In order to ascertain what I saw, the utterance has to be repeatable, so that I can recall what I saw when the insight has passed. The repeatability results from an idealization operated on the utterance. In fact an utterance cannot really be repeated on the same pitch, with the same tonal length, the same volume. When "thinking" of a past experience, I only imagine the words that formulate them, neglecting the actual differences in images formed at different times. Taking them to be ideally the same, I take them to have the same meaning.

I do have to repeat the formulation of my insight in order to represent what was seen in it when the insight passes with the passage of events and spectacles in the time of the world. But the formulation itself will pass from my representation of the things I have seen when a subsequent formulation conflicts with it. To reinstate my formulation, I shall have to resolve the conflict. I maintain that I did see a cobra by working out how the utterance "while working in the library, I saw a cobra" is compatible with subsequent utterances I make about what I saw there.

The idealization, abstracting from the concrete materiality of the utterance, that makes the utterance repeatable also makes it possible to abstract the formulation from the actual insight itself. The formulation can be recalled without reactivating the corresponding insight. From "I see that S is p," "S is p" can be retained in memory in the form of a belief. To believe that "S is p" is to maintain the insight as something that can be reactivated.

An utterance taken to be ideally repeatable in the absence of my insight which it originally formulated is ideally repeatable by others. Communication is taken to occur when, with an utterance another can repeat and whose meaning he or she can understand, the insight it formulates can be reactivated.

My formulation, which I can maintain only by committing myself to answer for it, will, when communicated, be subjected to contestation by subsequent statements others make. To maintain the truth of my own insights, I find myself elaborating justification for them in common language—in terms anyone can repeat and understand, with explanations anyone can judge and assent to. "I say that S is p" does not only record an insight; it is a pledge and a commitment. Communication becomes explanation and argument.

To maintain my own beliefs, I answer for them in communication with others by showing they are not inconsistent with what the others say. In doing so, I take the "S is p" that first formulated my insight and that I retain in my memory to be equivalent to the "S is p" that others have heard and retained and can see to be insightful. "I say that S is p" becomes "(It is said that) S is p." Credence in "S is p" can be maintained by me by turning into credence in the possibility of anyone seeing that "S is p." But then what it was that I saw, and maintained with a formulated belief, has been recast in an altered form. What I saw and what others can see are taken to be ideally the same.

There is then a triple idealization at work in communicating the insight that made it possible for me to say "I say that S is p." I—and the others—have to take the utterance "S is p" when repeated to be ideally the same, such that it can convey the same meaning. We have to take the insight that could be reactivated when the utterance is repeated by any of us to be ideally the same. And we have to take the state of affairs about which I had and the others could acquire an insight to be ideally the same. When the insight concerned a real state of affairs, it will not really be materially the same when that state of affairs is seen at another time or from another vantage point. The "S is p" that "is said" formulates not the concrete layout of the singular environment about the one who sees it, but abstracts certain features it designates as what anyone can see. Entities about which one could communicate formulations conveying credence in the same potential insights are constituted by idealization.

The statements communicated do not maintain the possibility of reactivating insights which are actual only in the first person singular, into situations that are each time singular. Instead, they maintain credence in the recurrent outlines of states of affairs and predicaments. The form in which an insight is retained and communicated displaces the form in which it is insightful.

The character of linguistic signs, which would all be universals, capable of designating only classes or series, does not explain the credence maintained in the recurrent character of what there is to be seen. One can use a linguistic formulation to recall a singular event in one's past. Communication by facial expressions, gestures, and manipulations can also make one take what one sees to be what anyone can see. But an insight need not be a singular act of a singular "I."

Our insights into the things we formulated in language are the work of our practical and perceptive, and also affective, powers. One finds oneself moved by the tone of the landscape and attracted to them and repelled by things, and one discovers and uncovers things by moving among them and manipulating them. Matters of public concern and personal interest direct scientific research. Scientific observation proceeds by manipulations, isolations, and experimentations, and employs instruments to refine substances and engineer verifications. Our insights into the meaning of the words we formulate call upon our ability to perceive and manipulate words we repeat and combine, and to do so while neglecting the material differences in their sounds when uttered, their visible forms when inscribed, or their images when we only "think" them.

We have learned from others what there is to see and how to look. We have learned to see what things are for by watching others use them or avoid them. Our interests and our indifference, our tastes and our repugnances have been shaped by those around us. When we begin to act, we "do what there is to be done." The way we do things—envision objectives and implements, grasp the environment significantly—we pass on to others who take their practicable situation to be equivalent and interchangeable with ours. We find we are doing what one does, before we shape actions on our own. We find we are saying "what one says." One takes up the talk before one speaks in one's own name.

Our gaze refracts off the substance of things to record outlines and patterns that recur. We stake out a manageable area in the practicable field and arrange things such that each day will layout equivalent tasks and implements. There is, Heidegger says, an unsleeping fear in this. There is a specific assurance in forming the trajectory of one's life into workdays that recur equivalent and interchangeable, and equivalent and interchangeable with those of others. One does not envision the singular without anxiety. The eyes that look closer to see the distinctive character of the layout about one sees the contingent and transitory character of the real. The hand that reaches out for the possibilities that are not those of anyone senses the risks and pitfalls in them. What covers over the outlying field of what is possible for anyone and outlines in relief what lies singularly at hand is the shadow of death singling one out. Fear of anxiety drives one to tear one's eyes from the singularity of the real in order to drift across recurrent outlines of things. One does not speak to articulate the singular predicament that sustains and threatens one's own unprecedented destiny, but speaks to communicate with the general lines of things and the recurrent patterns of events. One is speaking in order to not let one's voice and one's concerns die away; one is speaking out of fear of anxiety. Fear of anxiety is the unavowed force which motivates one to frame all one's utterances as "common sense," timeless verities, irrecusable commonplaces. One can find and one seeks not certainty but assurance in the formulas, in the talk that gets passed on.

I am anxious, I can sense the void, I can still feel the ground under my feet, I can sense possibilities for action, I doubt, I am thinking, I am—these would formulate insights I have into myself. I formulate these insights in order to be able to retain insight into myself. I exist, Descartes said, every time I *say* I exist. . . .

Self-consciousness is a need. It is the very articulation of our neediness—our mortality. But, Nietzsche writes, it articulates our mortality in the form of lacks and wants. The language of self-consciousness is a language of intentions, appetites, and volitions. They are articulated in general terms in order that others may understand them.[1]

It is only the "worst and most superficial part of ourselves" that can become conscious. For life is not the agitation of needs and wants in a material assemblage; life is force affirming itself and engendering energies over and beyond what is required to adjust to its environment and over and beyond the energies its absorbs. Life engenders excess forces which are felt in exhilaration and released in exuberance. Life's own forces are Apollonian and Dionysian, compulsions to produce visions the world does not give or require, to dream, and compulsions to move with nonteleological, gratuitous movements, to dance. Wants and needs and lacks are intermittent and surface occurrences, possible only because the core of life is plenitude and production of excess power.

If it is only our needs and wants that get articulated in the general terms of the language of self-consciousness, that is because the others understand and want to hear only our needs and lacks. Our needs and lacks are apprehended by the others as appeals to themselves, expressions of dependence on them, declarations of subservience, invitations to subjugation. The general terms of self-consciousness are herd-signals. It is through our needs and lacks that we appeal to the will in the others—the will to power in the others, the will to dominate.

It is in articulating ourselves as needs and lacks, in formulating ourselves as negativity, in becoming self-conscious, that we become servile. All the instincts of the servile are to make themselves weak; in all their talk they ask to be mastered. Expressing oneself in the (common) signs of language is itself what is debilitating and capitulating; self-consciousness is a disease.

In expressing oneself as a bundle of needs and cravings an individual makes himself common, and dependent, parasitical. At the same time one formulates the common representation of the universe in the value dichotomies of good and bad, positive and negative, resources and lacks, devaluing all that is ephemeral, transitory, fragmentary, enigmatic, all that eludes the rapacious nets of common reason and utility.

To find the word that can be true, the speech acts that reveal, it is necessary, Heidegger says, to withdraw from the talk into reticence[2]— into the silence that answers not to another, always there, but to the silence of death, even now imminent. The approach of death silences the solicitations that general possibilities address to one, and makes one hearken to one's own singular situation, which solicits one's own powers. Out of this silence a speech can begin that articulates one's own singular situation, for oneself. This speech— and not the common talk articulating the general lines of the world—can be true, for reality is in the singular. Articulating possibilities that answer to or are deaf to my own powers, this speech of one's own singularizes the speaker who says "I."

For Heidegger what makes a speech act true is not a personal intuition conceived as an immediate grasp of the given. The uncovering that breaks through the leveling and idealizing interpretations in what "one says" to articulate what is really possible and is is a temporal process, enlisting various approaches and manipulations, including the guidelines of propositions already fixed in the common language. What is essential is that an agency be set up that commits itself to this work. The "I" is this agency, this responsibility. Taking what is said and passed about as subject to question, I answer by answering to the solicitations my practicable environment addresses singularly to me. Such are speech acts that are "my own" (*eigen*), speech acts in which a sphere of ownness, an *Eigentlichkeit*, constitutes itself.

The anxiety which senses the death coming for me measures, in the field of possibilities ahead which are possibilities for anyone, the confines of the possibilities that are possible for me. Anxiety senses that others are different, stationed before tasks and concerns which are not for me. I no longer view them as instances, equivalent to and interchangeable with myself, of anonymous diagrams of actions, figures of a life that goes on without end. I sense the others in their mortality. To sense another acting in another expanse of possibilities delimited by a menace of death which does not figure in my field of possibilities and my future is to see him living in the trajectory of another time, extending from his birth to the death. This nonsimultaneity, this deferral of his death relative to my own makes each moment present to him nonsimultaneous with the moment at which I am present. In this deferral and this distance, the other, another one like myself, is different.

This vision is a solicitude, for the first and best thing I can do for another, if I care about him or her, is to deliver him or her over to his or her own tasks by resolutely pursuing my own. What speech would communicate this solicitude? The care for the different one is not simply marked by indexical terms: "here," "yonder," "I," "you," attached to words whose meaning, in what I say and in what the other says, is equivalent and interchangeable. It is elaborated in a speech that responds to the different one by articulating the possibilities in my own situation addressed singularly to my own powers.

Each of the acts that surge forth from the plenitude of one's nature is unutterably singular, Nietzsche writes, though when it is formulated in the language—the herd-signals—of self-consciousness they no longer seem to be. Conscience is the proximity to one's own nature, Apollonian and Dionysian, whose needs and wants are only superficial and intermittent, whose compulsion is to discharge the excess life continually generates in dreams and dances.

When conductors and performers first saw the score of the *Missa Solemnis*, they thought Beethoven had been deaf so long that he no longer realized that no human voice could sing the notes he had written. Before the end of his life, they finally gave Beethoven an orchestra and singers to train. When the performance was over and Beethoven's hands and baton were still, the audience rose to their feet applauding and shouting their acclaim, but Beethoven did not turn around to bow. After a long time, the soprano soloist moved to him and gently turned him around so that he could see the enthusiasm of the crowd. What the crowd saw then were his eyes streaming with tears. Not tears of grief that he could not hear what he had composed and conducted—for he heard all its grandeur inwardly: tears of joy and gratitude that he had been given a power so grandiose and so sacred.

For Beethoven to know himself is to know there is a power to make the world resound with music which, if he did not compose it, would never be heard; conscience is the proximity maintained to this power. It can nowise be formulated in the language of self-consciousness. It is known and expressed—by others as by himself—in the very composing of this music. It is only in the tears that flowed from his face that he knew he had the singular power to compose the *Missa Solemnis*.

In this man there is a power to run as no one can run, to run like deer run, with a grace that the stopwatches and numbers do not record. In this woman there is a power to be a mother as no one can be a mother, to squander kisses and caresses over this criminal or over this deformed orphan child no one else could love. The legs that trace this run across the savannah and the forest, the kisses and caresses that rain across the hills and valleys of this flesh, are the inscription of singular lives.

Yet language too does not only communicate, but reveals. The general terms with which one articulates a singular event and a response to it designate, in one's memory, that singularity and recall it. The singular one, Heidegger believes, also discovers his own singular powers in articulating them in language. The words of language do not capture singular powers all at once; they maintain one's own attention on them by a never-ending elaboration. But what makes one's speech one's own is not simply that with the words of anyone one composes combinations no one else has put together. Language, Heidegger says, also determines the ways in which one lets the environment concern one— one's moods. One's moods reveal where one is and how one is. One's mood, and the weight of the environment felt on a singular here, are conveyed in language not so much by the meaning and referents of the words, but by their tone—by the emphasis, rhythm, cadences, and silences of one's speech.

This is why Nietzsche says that a philosopher who has a conscience writes a philosophy that must sing. Like Beethoven finds himself in the *Missa Solemnis* upon which he has squandered all his forces, Nietzsche finds himself in books that contain not only ideas no one has composed with words which are the words of everyone, but words that chant and dance.

Nietzsche finds, besides the language of self-consciousness, a language of self-consecration. The joyous exclamations "How happy I am!" "How healthy I am!" "How beautiful I am!" were the inventions with which a sovereign individual consecrates and enhances his or her own superabundance of being and vitality.[3] They function not to record and retain a passing insight, but to intensify a present and future power. Evolving from the chant of insects and birds, these intonations gave their meaning to all the noble and ennobling words of language. Intensifying the gratuitous radiance and rhythm of superabundant life, speech chants and dances in them.

These noble and ennobling words are repeatable, by oneself and by others. They can communicate what I feel to another who has been driven, by the forces of his own feeling, to utter these exclamations. What communicates in them is not their semantic form, distinguished by semantic markers within a system of other signifiers. What communicates is the tone in which they are uttered, the pacing, the cadence, the place and time in which they are uttered, breaking the sequence of indications and designations, appeals and demands.

A language can be used not to convey, but to take the place of, reality. The language of self-consciousness covers over the deep and positive reality of life. But once the vocabulary of self-consciousness has been constituted, it can, like any accumulation, be squandered. The rhetoric of supplication, that of orators, preachers, and psychologists introduces an artistry on the material of self-consciousness. For one whose conscience keeps him or her in proximity with the deepest and best part of himself or herself, all the rhetoric of self-consciousness is fiction. It can give rise, in writers of fiction, to a spiritual—pneumatic, witty—expenditure.

The language of the world can also be squandered, and die away in the rumble of nature.

In this epoch of the end of ideology and the third, information, revolution, the conversion of insightful and significant utterances into excitants of needs is the pilot industry of postindustrial, postindustrious capitalism. It seizes upon every communicable utterance—the axioms of science that trigger intellectual recognition, the "Aha!" that greets pleasures, the yeses that incite cravings—to code ever more deeply individuals as grasping hands and gaping mouths.

But there is another relapse into babble, into infantilism, that occurs in human communication reduced to garrulousness. Human voices that were raised to fix and retain the truth of the world and answer for it ramble and reverberate. One finds oneself speaking only for the pleasure of hearing oneself talk, for the carnality of the formulations indefinitely repeated, for the rhythms and the rumble, for the warmth and moistness of the breath. Sometimes one finds then that, like the one that opens his house to the passerby and speaks meaningless conventions without query or truth, one's voice is a murmur that delineates and condenses a zone of intimacy and hospitality.

And sometimes one finds then that one's voice which no longer fixes insights into things and delineates the ways of the world, rumbles on in the undifferentiated, unbounded expanses of the light, of the atmosphere, in which the carpentry of the world is suspended and shimmers and drifts. Joining the incantations of the frogs in the swamps, the celestial birds, the insects swarming in the night. A voice in which the forms of things dissolve as it drifts into the elemental. And babble resounds with another truth.

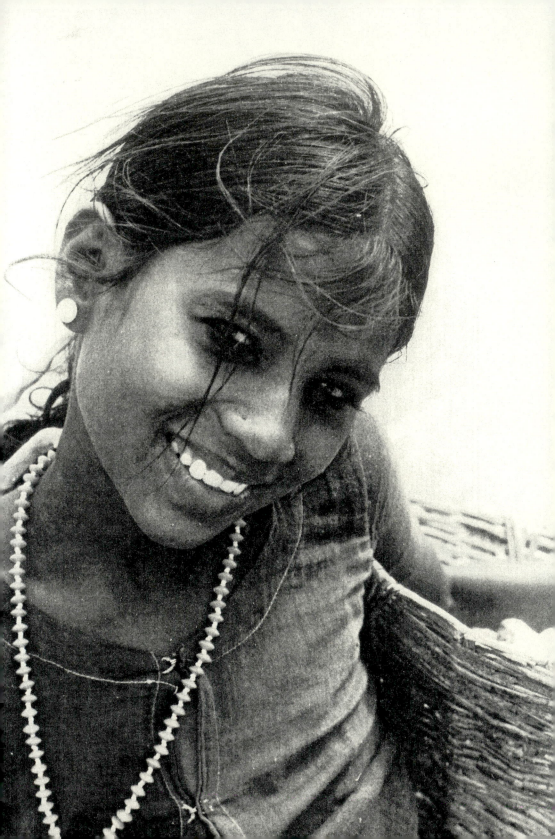

8

◆

Surface Effects

From one end to the other of this human life which is our lot, the consciousness of the paucity of stability, even of the profound lack of all true stability, liberates the enchantment of laughter. As if this life suddenly passed from an empty and sad solidity to the happy contagion of warmth and of light, to the free tumult which the waters and the air communicate to one another: flashes and the rebounding of laughter follow the first opening, the permeability of a dawning smile. If a group of people laugh at an absent-minded gesture, or at a sentence revealing an absurdity, there passes within them a current of intense communication. Each isolated existence emerges from itself by means of the image betraying the error of immutable isolation. It emerges from itself in a sort of easy flash; it opens itself at the same time to the contagion of a wave which rebounds, for those who laugh, together become like the waves of the sea—there no longer exists between them any partition as long as the laughter lasts; they are no more separate then are two waves, but their unity is as undefined, as precarious as that of the agitation of the waters.[1]

Communication ceases to be the circulation of information and the exchange of the equivalent when I find myself not only different from the others, but contested by them. It ceases to be subjection and domination when it is gratuitous celebration in laughter and blessings.

Appeals and demands are formulated in the vocative and imperative forms of grammar. They contest what is, require something other than what is. Communicated to me, their meaning reconstituted by my understanding, they are but formulations which I can take as maxims or programs I can use to diagram my acts. I will do so when I understand that what another sees as required, from his or her situation in the practicable layout, is what is required in the practicable environment about me. This understanding first understands the practicable field about me as equivalent and interchangeable with that of any other. To take a maxim to be required everywhere and imposed on everyone is to take it as a law.

The law, in which what is imperative is formulated, is other than what is and other than what I am. But in formulating it, I represent it to myself, where, as a representation, it is maintained by my own representational faculty. Thus, in Kant's words, I am subject to the law of which I am myself the legislator. But to find myself subject to it is to not only understand its formulation, but to feel its imperative force. The imperative force is not something I represent; it is given in the faculty of feeling, in the sentiment of respect.

What is it that I feel in the sentiment of respect? I feel, Kant says, the imperative force of what has the form of law. I feel the force of the imperative for the universal and the necessary, for reason. Understanding without content is empty. I feel the rationally understandable world as a force weighing on me and requiring me. I feel the pressure of a world in which the environments about perceiving and acting individuals are equivalent and interchangeable.

But it also happens that another singles me out with an appeal and a demand that is his or her own. Inasmuch as the other singles me out and addresses me, he or she stands apart from me and stands apart too from the series in which I situated him when observing and identifying him or her. He or she is you, unidentified, unclassified, unformed, addressed with a pronoun that is not a stand-in for a name.

What I understand is not simply a formulation whose meaning I reconstitute, interpreting it out of the context of the order of my reasons, according to my own codes. I find the ordering advance of my understanding of the environment interrupted and disputed. And I feel that what the other says binds me; I feel its imperative force. I feel the other—other than me, other than the others—as a force that holds me and to which I am subject. In being singled out by the other, I respond not as an another one, but in my own name, as I.

The experience of finding oneself under an imperative is then not only an immemorial or a priori state of finding one's understanding subjected to the weight of a rationally ordered world to be understood and dealt with practically. It is an event, which occurs when another faces me—an intermittent and surface event.

To face me is to appeal to me and to lay a demand on me—if only that I interrupt what I am doing to offer a sign or word of greeting. To face me is to ask and require something of me—a response in my own name that answers to what the other formulates.

Jean-Luc Nancy says that the imperative belongs to language, is possible only in language.[2] The very term was invented by Immanuel Kant. But language is a second-order conventionalization of the expressive body. It can no more condense in its formulations all that appeals and demands in that body than it can tell all that one sees, touches, and feels as one walks in the forest.

The other appeals and requires me with a look, a gesture, a pressure of the hand, a shiver on the skin.

In responding to what the other asks and demands, I formulate what I have seen and understood. But the production of a discourse in the terms of a common language, a body of statements reciprocally affirmed, is not the telos of the face-to-face encounter, any more than self-consciousness is of life. The other requires of me what I myself have seen, touched, felt, and the resources of my lucidity, my tact and tenderness, my mobility and repose.

If the imperative is a phenomenal event, it is not to be described as something realized in an ideal order into which intellectual intuition has insight. What makes the imperative appear as a fact is not an ideal, norm, or standard that would subsist apart from the observable environment. The phenomenal apparition of the imperative is not to be described as something realized in the plenitude and perfection of an exemplary being in the world. For Kant to respect the other is to respect the law—more exactly, the imperative for law— at work in him, which binds me also. It is to see his actions and words diagramming what reason requires anyone must do in a practicable field such as his. But for Kant it is on my own understanding that I feel the force of the imperative for law, and the phenomenal appearance of the other is only a schema of the imperative for law whose force I know inwardly.

Emmanuel Levinas finds the encounter with the imperative in the sensory event of someone facing me in the nakedness and vulnerability of his or her eyes on which the forms of the environment leave no trace; in the emptiness of his or her hands that gesture to me, forming and deforming themselves in the void, grasping nothing, turned to me; in the stumblings and the avid discomfited silences that break through the conventional garb and rhetorical adornment of his or her sentences, in the insubstantiality of the voice that dies away as soon as they are uttered. In them the voice that formulates words, the look that holds my eyes, the hands that reach out for mine do not only indicate and inform, but appeal and demand. These fleeting and insubstantial surface effects do not reveal the solidity and inner composition of a depth, but hollow out wants and lacks, vulnerability and susceptibility.

The appeal and demand of the other surfaces on the skin, which is not a hide, camouflage, or container, but a surface of exposure. The bared skin upon which expressions form and dissolve, engulfed in the evidence of impressionability and vulnerability, exposes the sensibility of the other. The skin which supports the signs of an alien intention and alien moods effaces them in its quivering susceptibility and in the wrinkles of its aging and mortality. The skin, weighed down with wounds, scars, and wrinkles exposes the vulnerability and mortality of the other.

The imperative force is not something I represent; it is that to which I find myself subjected. It is not in representing to myself the figure of the other, who presents himself or herself to me, but in making contact with his or her look, touch, and voice that I feel the imperative force of an alien appeal and demand. There is immediacy in this contact with a sensory figure I am prevented from observing.

One can indeed look at and touch the skin of another like the surface of a thing it contains and whose inner constitution it reveals. One can see, in an aesthetic contemplation, the skin as materializing a form and extending a coloration that holds the light. But when one makes contact with it, with the look that grazes it or the hand that caresses it, one touches the skin as the surface of exposure, whereby the other is exposed to the harsh reality of things and to the egoism and violence in me. The skin is a surface of sensitivity and susceptibility. The other in baring his or her skin exposes his or her vulnerability to pain, to wounds and outrage, exposes his or her mortality. One's gaze and touch sense it in the tremblings of pleasure that die away, the anxieties of pain that agitate those surfaces. One senses the vulnerability in the wrinkles with which aging inscribes the pressure of imminent death. One senses it in the lassitude and torpor into which the expressions he or she addresses to me sink.

To make contact with this surface of sensitivity and susceptibility is to be excited by its pleasure and afflicted with its pain. This pleasure and pain are not observed from a distance; they are felt immediately in one's own sensitivity and susceptibility. When the other looks at me I no longer observe his eyes; I feels his gaze in feeling my gaze turned on him softening. When the others hails me and gestures to me, my hands halt in mid-air, detached from my working posture and my projects; I feel their grip invaded by tact and tenderness. When the other greets me, and questions me, I feel the hesitations and silences that invade my voice, making of my convictions and affirmations questions put to him or her. The look that grazes and the touch that caresses the bared skin of her face and hands, while recording its color and elasticity, is troubled by the torments and pleasures that surface on it.

The other in whom the imperative makes an appearance is not an ideal, norm, or standard. He or she is not the sage, hero, and saint that would be the material figure of morality. His or her imperative alterity is not realized in the plenitude and perfection of an exemplary being in the world. It appears in surface effects of susceptibility and destitution, vulnerability and mortality. Alterity weighs on us in the words of foreigners and of those without scientific culture, in the nonsense of children and the laughter of adults and nonwisdom of the aged, in the gaze and outstretched hand of the sick and the dying.

But the imperative phenomenon is not a simple compound of being and nothingness, of plenitude and need. The face is not a surface that presents signs that signify an absence. The wants and needs of the other are positive as an imperative force. The face is the phenomenal event of what is other than being but not nothingness. Levinas introduces alterity as a third category irreducible to being and nothingness.

What can one say about the alterity revealed in the you that addresses me? Only, Levinas says, that it is separation itself, beyond being, metaphysical. It is the infinite separation or unending removal by which the other stands apart from the substance of his body inasmuch as I can take hold of it and comprehend it, stands apart from every representation with which I seek to comprehend him, by contesting that representation, or by assenting to it. The face is the trace left of a departure. The other is separation or sacredness in the singular. "You" is the pronoun put in place of what never has a name or identity—like the God of monotheism, Levinas says, who is not a figure of the sacred, or a being to whom categories can be predicated. The other that faces me faces in the image and likeness of God.

This train of thought, however, runs the risk of undermining the essential contribution of Levinas's phenomenology of the face. Alterity described as separation, absence, absoluteness, transcendence, and infinity or infinition formulates a negative metaphysics. This metaphysics is the counterpart of Levinas's positivist phenomenology, which finds no appeal and demand in the earth and skies, plants and animals, and describes sensory things as substances whose contours offer them to removal, usage, and appropriation.

Describing more closely the appeal and demand with which the other faces makes it possible for us to avoid this negative metaphysics and determine the alterity of the other in the *physis* that is reality and apparition.

The other who reaches out to me reaches out for the skills and resources of my hands. But he does not ask that I take over his tasks for him. She asks of my hands the diagram of the operations her hands are trying to perform and requires the assistance of my forces lest hers be wanting. But the other asks first for terrestrial support. The fatigue, the vertigo, the homelessness in his body appeal for support from my earthbound body which has the sense of this terrain to give. If, while extending my skills to her tasks I do not offer this support, the other will prefer to work out the ways and the operations on her own by trial and error.

The other asks not only for cooperation, but contact. In the clasped handshake with which we greet one another and set out each to his or her own tasks, the other seeks the warmth and the tact that the fingers and palm of my hand extend.

The other, in approaching me, appeals for information from me, appeals to me to turn to him or her the forms my eyes have illuminated, the fields my understanding has clarified. But his or her eyes look first for the vivacity and delight of the light in my eyes and the shadows and darkness my eyes harbor with care. Should I turn to him dark eyes he or she will seek rather in books the formulas and the information.

His or her words, which I understand because they are the words of my own tongue, ask for information and indications. They ask for a response that will be responsible, will give reasons for its reasons, that will be a commitment to answer for what it answers. But they first greet me, appealing for responsiveness. His words seek out a voice voluble and spiritual, a voice whose orders and coherence and direction are interrupted, of itself, by hesitations, redundancies, silences, questioning the other by questioning itself. In the very explanation and instruction the other seeks, she seeks her own voice in my silences and my questions. If my voice is not responsive to this quest, he or she will seek in manuals the answers to his or her perplexities.

The separation, absence, absoluteness, transcendence, and infinity or infinition with which Levinas characterizes negatively the otherness of the other is revealed positively in the dark light that refracts from his eyes to solicit the light in my eyes, in the resonance held back which seeks its voice in my silences and questions, in the warmth and susceptibility of his or her bare hands disengaged from the things to reach out for the tact and tenderness in my hands. The face of another is a surface of the elemental, the place where the elemental addresses, appeals and requires the involution in enjoyment which makes my eyes luminous, my hands warm, my posture supportive, my voice voluble and spiritual, my face ardent.

Human bodies are not opaque material masses whose axis of position and diagram of movement we scan and interpret. They move in the environment engendering profiles and telescoping images of themselves, casting shadows, sending off rustlings and echoes, leaving traces and stains. The presence of someone in the world is a track soon effaced left in the streets and the fields, warmth left in the hands of others and in the winds, sweat left on tools and chairs, a voice others have carried away or that is lost in the night. Those we call solid and self-sufficient, on the move, making a name for themselves, are discharging their energies in enterprises that will endure but that absorb and render anonmyous all the human thought, imagination, and effort that go into them. The one that singles me out addresses to me the sensitivity, susceptibility, vulnerability, and mortality of his or her presence in the world, to require from someone equally exposed and insubstantial light, ardor, warmth, and support.

The material things too do not lie naked and impassive in a space through which a transparent and innocuous time flows. They occupy and extend space generating perspectival deformations of their surfaces, scattering their colors in the light and their images on surrounding things. They project hints and lures and leave traces. They prolong the entry of the present sending echoes and heralds of themselves in waves of time. In doing so they can be found and can be real. They also cast shadows and form screens and phosphorescent veils; their surfaces double up into facades. They generate halos and phantasmal reflections of themselves. The volumes shaped with shadows, the refracted colors mixed with reflections, the omens and lures, the halos and the mirages make the things visible and are the visibility the things engender. The rumble and echoes that make everything that is resound, the odors they broadcast, the contours with which they receive one another and slip across one another and the hollows of things with which they churn the wind and gather the rain, and the night they cast about their luminous outcroppings belong to the reality of things and make their presence about us real.

The things are not only structures with closed contours that lend themselves to manipulation and whose consistency constrains us. They lure and threaten us, support and orient and disorient us, sustain and debilitate us, direct us and calm us. They enrapture us with their sensuous substances and also with their luminous surfaces and their phosphorescent facades, their halos, their radiance and their resonances.

Nietzsche denounces the self-consciousness in which I formulate myself as a bundle of wants and needs and make myself dependent and servile. He denounces the pity that sees the frailty and vulnerability of another and the compassion contaminated by his or her suffering. He acknowledges the celebration with which a strong and joyous vitality consecrates the nobility of those one hears exclaiming "How happy I am!" "How healthy I am!" "How beautiful I am!" He proclaims a communication beyond good and evil, which celebrates the artists who work with the most precious clay and oil, their own flesh and blood. Not only their words, but their gestures and their silences speak or chant. He calls for not a face to face confrontation that appeals and demands, but a communication of the joyous in words of consecration, chant, and laughter.

But bodies do not occupy their spot in space and time, filling it to capacity, such that their beauty would be statuesque. We do not see bodies whose form and colors are held by concepts we recognize or reconstitute. We do not see bodies in their own integrity and inner coherence. Strength does not consist in force contained, health does not consist in purity and integrity in a body that is porous and where the generation of excess energies is expenditure and decomposition.

The face of another that addresses me and that appeals and demands is a dispersion of surface effects that make my eyes luminous, my hands warm, my posture supportive, my voice voluble and spiritual, my face ardent. In the poverty and destitution, vulnerability and mortality of flesh are all the laughter and blessings that resounds on human faces.

Jean Genet is struck by the cool eyes of a feyadee youth on the way to die in Jordan. He is moved by the narrow lives of the Palestinian women in the camps, their age-old memory as if made up of the stitches in their ancient embroidered gowns: the sum of many brief, tiny memories laid end to end, so that the women know when to buy thread, to sew on a few buttons, patch the seat of a pair of trousers or go back to the shop for some salt, and to endure the forgetting of past sufferings.[3] An old Palestinian woman said to him: "To have been dangerous for a thousandth of a second, to have been handsome for a thousandth of a thousandth of a second, to have been that, or happy or something, and then to rest—what more can one want?"[4] For fourteen years he sought in love marks on a thin, suspicious face, a few grey hairs, and some smears of henna on a withered skin.[5]

A face speaks blessings by the fire in its eyes and the vivacity of its organs, the spiritedness of its substance, the exceptional expressiveness of the movements that form and fade across it, the harmony or vigor of its contours and tones. Not so much the force available in it to effect changes on the things as the somber light that glows on its bared surfaces and in the involuntary grace of its gestures makes us see another's bodily presence as a blessing in the midst of things. His or her hands leave blessings in brief embraces and light touches that were not made to steady our hand. The ardor and vivacity of his or her eyes make the things touched briefly by them flare.

In the rigor and solidity of another's words we divine a coherent implantation in the wide world. It is not in the rigor and coherence of her information and her convictions, not in her wisdom but in her wit, or the wisdom of her wit, the rhythm of her repetitions of stock phrases, the occasional odd combination of words, the poetry of her nonsense, and the timbre and radiance of her voice and her silences that we recognize the singularity of another. The vivacity of his mind speaking an idiolect of clandestine allusions, private jokes, whimsical taxonomies, perverse explanations makes the landscape sparkle with laughter. "In the middle of the night, in the middle of the bed, between the sheets, an almost wordless language, or one that makes words mean their opposite is forged between two lovers," Jean Genet writes. "Wherever it occurs, this nocturnal language between two lovers creates a night. They take refuge in it even among a thousand or a hundred thousand others, who may have held their noses at the moisture of their reunion."[6]

Words of consecration do not function to fix a form that can be maintained. They function to intensify a surge of vitality generating excess energies. Their expression sends forth those energies in expenditure without return. The one who exclaims "How happy I am!" already catches sight of friends and strangers, trees and skies upon whom to discharge the warmth and light of his happiness. The one who hears that exclamation feels a surge of happiness in himself straining to release itself. They are traces of departure, departing traces.

Notes

CHAPTER 1: We Mortals

1. Martin Heidegger, *Being and Time*, trans. John Macquarrie and Edward Robinson (New York: Harper & Row, 1962), pp. 317–23.
2. Ibid., pp. 163–68.
3. Martin Heidegger, *What is Metaphysics?* trans. David Farrell Krell in David Farrell Krell, ed., *Martin Heidegger, Basic Writings* (New York: Harper & Row), 1977), pp. 95–112.
4. Martin Heidegger, *Being and Time*, pp. 300–304, 309–11.
5. Ibid., pp. 346–47.
6. Martin Heidegger, *Poetry, Language, Thought*, trans. Albert Hofstadter (New York: Harper & Row, 1971), pp. 159–61.
7. Heidegger, *Being and Time*, p. 434.
8. Aristotle, *Nichomachean Ethics*, trans. Martin Ostwald (Indianapolis: Bobbs-Merrill, 1962) pp. 68–77.

CHAPTER 2: The World as a Whole

1. Martin Heidegger, *Being and Time*, trans. John Macquarrie and Edward Robinson (New York: Harper & Row, 1962).
2. *Being and Time* had put aside the word "thing" to describe intramundane entities. (pp. 96–97) "The Origin of the Work of Art" rejected it as a general term with no unified meaning, of which natural beings, implements, and artworks, and even young girls and God would be specifications. (Martin Heidegger, *Poetry, Language, Thought*, trans. Albert Hofstadter (New York: Harper & Row, 1971), pp. 20–22.) The essay "The Thing," however, finds that etymologically the term means not an assemblage, but an assembler, and designates as things cross and crown (ritual objects), bench and plow (implements), heron and roe (natural beings). (Ibid., pp. 174–75, 182).
3. Materiality figures as reliability—materialization of serviceability. It is sensed through the form.
4. Heidegger, "The Origin of the Work of Art," p. 35.
5. Martin Heidegger, "On the Essence of Truth," trans. John Sallis in David Farrell Krell, Martin Heidegger, *Basic Writings* (New York: Harper & Row, 1977), pp. 135–37.
6. Heidegger, *Being and Time*, p. 434.
7. Maurice Merleau-Ponty, *The Visible and the Invisible*, trans. Alphonso Lingis (Evanston: Northwestern University Press, 1968), p. 237.
8. Heidegger, *Poetry, Language, Thought*, p. 178.
9. Heidegger, *Being and Time*, pp. 434–35.

10. "Scarcely an object, [the glassy plastic drinking cup] is so superbly universal Hegel might have halloed at it. Made of a substance found nowhere in nature, manufactured by processes equally unnatural and strange, it is the complete and expert artifact. Then packaged in sterilized stacks as though it weren't a thing at all by itself, this light, translucent emptiness is so utterly identical to the other items in its package, the other members of its class, it might almost be space. Sloganless— it has no message—often not even the indented hallmark of its maker. It is an abstraction acting as a glass, and resists individuation perfectly, because you can't crimp its rim or write on it or poke it full of pencil holes—it will shatter first, rather than submit—so there is no way, after a committee meeting, a church sup or reception (its ideal locales), to know one from the other, as it won't discolor, stain, craze, chip, but simply safeguards the world from its contents until both the flat Coke or cold coffee and their cup are disposed of. It is a decendental object. It cannot have a history. It has disappeared entirely into its function. It is completely what it does, except that what it does, it does as a species. Of itself it provides no experience, and scarcely of its kind. Even a bullet gets uniquely scarred. Still, this *shotte*, this *nebech*, is just as much a cultural object, and just as crystalline in its way, as our golden bowl, and is without flaws, and costs nothing, and demands nothing, and is one of the ultimate wonders of the universe of *dreck*— the world of neutered things. It *is* perfect. That is Arnold's word.

   "Nevertheless, the perfections of this plain clear plastic up perversely deny it perfection. Since it is nothing but its use, its existence is otherwise ignored. It is not worth a rewash. it is not worth another look, a feel, a heft. It has been desexed. Thus indifference is encouraged. Consumption is encouraged. Convenience is encouraged. Castoffs are multiplied, and our world is already full of the unwanted and used up. Its rim lies along the lip like the edge of a knife. That quality is also ignored and insensitivity encouraged. It is a servant, but it has none of the receptivity of artistic material, and in that sense it does not serve; its absences are everywhere. Since, like an overblown balloon, it has as much emptiness as it can take, it is completely its shape, and because it totally contains, it is estranged from what it holds. Thus dissociation is encouraged. Poured into such a vessel, wine moans for a certain moment, and then is silent; its color pales, its bouquet faces, it becomes pop; yet there is a pallid sadness in its modest mimicry of the greater goblets, in its pretense to perfect nothingness, in its ordinary evil, since it is no Genghis Khan, or Coriolanus, but a discreet and humble functionary, simply doing its job as it has been designed and directed to do, like the other members of the masses, and disappearing with less flutter than leaves." William H. Gass, *Habitations of the Word* (New York: Simon & Schuster, 1985), pp. 204–205.
11. Heidegger, "The Thing," in *Poetry, Language, Thought*, p. 182.
12. Emmanuel Levinas, *Totality and Infinity*, trans. Alphonso Lingis, 2nd ed. (The Hague, Martinus Nijhoff, 1979), p. 133.
13. Ibid., p. 167.
14. Emmanuel Levinas, *Existence and Existents*, trans. Alphonso Lingis (The Hague: Martinus Nijhoff, 1978), p. 29.
15. Heidegger, *Being and Time*, p. 173.
16. Ibid., p. 175.
17. Ibid.
18. Heidegger, *Being and Time*, p. 100–101. This is not essentially changed when, in the

later theory of the Fourfold, the heavens are described as the region of the changing light and seasons which bring forth what grows of itself and makes them visible and accessible in the interplay of light and shadow. *Poetry, Language, Thought*, pp. 149, 178.
19. Martin Heidegger, "Thinking Building Dwelling" trans. Alfred Hofstadter, in Martin Heidegger, *Poetry, Language, Thought*, pp. 145–61.

CHAPTER 3: Imperatives

1. Maurice Merleau-Ponty, *Phenomenology of Perception*, trans. Colin Smith (London: Routledge & Kegan Paul, 1986), p. 4.
2. Ibid., pp. 299–327.
3. Maurice Merleau-Ponty, *The Visible and the Invisible*, trans. Alphonso Lingis (Evanston: Northwestern University Press, 1969), p. 8.
4. Merleau-Ponty, *Phenomenology of Perception*, pp. 243–327.
5. Ibid., pp. 327–34.
6. Ibid., pp. 374–77. *The Visible and the Invisible*, pp. 40–42.
7. Merleau-Ponty, *Phenomenology of Perception*, pp. 280–98.
8. Martin Heidegger, *Kant and the Problem of Metaphysics*, trans. Richard Taft (Bloomington, Indiana University Press, 1990), p. 19.
9. *Phenomenology of Perception*, pp. xix–xxi.
10. Ibid., pp. 139–42.
11. Ibid., pp. 208–11.
12. Ibid., pp. 251–53.
13. Merleau-Ponty, *The Visible and the Invisible*, p. 8.
14. Merleau-Ponty, *Phenomenology of Perception*, pp. 67–72.
15. Ibid., p. 327.
16. Ibid., pp. 56–59.
17. Ibid., pp. 56–62.
18. Maurice Merleau-Ponty, *The Structure of Behavior*, trans. (Boston: Beacon, 1959).

CHAPTER 4: The Body Postured and Dissolute

1. Maurice Merleau-Ponty, *Phenomenology of Perception*, trans. Colin Smith (London: Routledge & Kegan Paul and New Jersey: Humanities, 1986).
2. Sigmund Freud, *Civilization and Its Discontents*, trans. James Strachey, *The Standard Edition of the Complete Psychological Works of Sigmund Freud*, Vol. XXI (London: Hogarth Press, 1961), p. 82.
3. Sigmund Freud, *Three Essays on the Theory of Sexuality*, trans. James Strachey, *The Standard Edition of the Complete Psychological Works of Sigmund Freud*, vol. VII (London: Hogarth Press, 1953), p. 203.
4. Ibid., p. 61.
5. Sigmund Freud, *Beyond the Pleasure Principle*, trans. James Strachey, *The Standard Edition of the Complete Psychological Works of Sigmund Freud*, vol. 18, p. 20.
6. Ibid., p. 39.
7. Ibid., pp. 39–40.
8. Ibid., pp. 90, 41.
9. Gilles Deleuze and Félix Guattari, *Anti-Oedipus*, trans. M. Seem, R. Hurley, & H. R. Lane (New York: Viking: 1977), p. 294.
10. Jean Baudrillard, *Seduction*, trans. Brian Singer (New York: St. Martin's Press, 1990).

CHAPTER 5: Face-to-Face

1. Emmanuel Levinas, *Totality and Infinity*, trans. Alphonso Lingis (The Hague: Martinus Nijhoff, 1979), pp. 35–40.
2. Ibid., p. 39.
3. Ibid., p. 74.
4. Ibid., pp. 75, 199–200.
5. Emmanuel Levinas, *Otherwise than Being or Beyond Essence*, trans. Alphonso Lingis (The Hague: Martinus Nijhoff, 1981), pp. 75–76.
6. Emmanuel Levinas, *Collected Philosophical Papers*, pp. 123–124.
7. Martin Heidegger, *Being and Time*, trans. John Macquarrie and Edward Robinson (New York: Harper & Row, 1962), pp. 330–31.

CHAPTER 6: Sensuality and Sensitivity

1. Martin Heidegger, *Being and Time*, trans. John Macquarrie and Edward Robinson (New York: Harper & Row, 1962), p. 177.
2. Ibid., p. 174.
3. Ibid., p. 175.
4. Ibid., pp. 235–37, 383ff.
5. Ibid., pp. 304–311, 341–48.
6. Emmanuel Levinas, *Totality and Infinity*, trans. Alphonso Lingis (The Hague: Martinus Nijhoff, 1979), pp. 110–112.
7. Ibid., pp. 110–121, 127–130.
8. Emmanuel Levinas, *Otherwise than Being or Beyond Essence*, trans. Alphonso Lingis (The Hague: Martinus Nijhoff, 1981), pp. 75–81.
9. Martin Heidegger, *An Introduction to Metaphysics*, trans. Ralph Manheim (Garden City, New York: Doubleday, 1961).
10. Heidegger, *Being and Time*, pp. 319–21.
11. Levinas, *Totality and Infinity*, pp. 197–201.
12. Levinas, *Otherwise than Being or Beyond Essence*, pp. 81–89.

CHAPTER 7: What is Passed Over in Communication

1. Friedrich Nietzsche, *The Gay Science*, trans. Walter Kaufmann (New York: Vintage, 1974), ¶ 354.
2. Ibid., p. 208.
3. Friedrich Nietzsche, *On the Genealogy of Morals*, trans. Walter Kaufmann (New York: Vintage, 1969), pp. 28–30.

CHAPTER 8: Surface Effects

1. Georges Bataille, *Inner Experience*, trans. Leslie Anne Boldt (New YOrk: State University of New York Press, 1988), pp. 95–96.
2. Jean-Luc Nancy, *L'impératif catégorique* (Paris: Flammarion).
3. Jean Genet, *Prisoner of Love*, trans. Barbara Bray (Hanover and London: Wesleyan University Press, 1992), p. 229.
4. Ibid., p. 234.
5. Ibid., p. 331.
6. Ibid., p. 329.

Index

———◆———